Free and Easy

Traditional Chinese Gynecology For American Women

D1604224

by

Bob Flaws

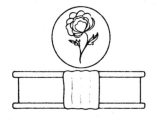

Blue Poppy Press

Published by:

Blue Poppy Press
1775 Linden Ave.
Boulder, CO 80304
(303) 442-0796

First Edition October, 1986
Second Edition June, 1990

ISBN 0-936185-05-8

The information in this book is given in good faith. However, the translators and publisher cannot be held responsible for any error or omission. Nor can they be held in any way responsible for treatment given on the basis of information contained int his book. The publishers make this information available to English readers fo scholarly and research purposes only.

The publishers do not advocate nor endorse self-medication by laypersons. Chinese medicine is a professional medicine. Laypersons interested in availing themselves of the treatment described in this book should seek out a qualified professional practitioner of Chinese medicine.

PREFACE TO
SECOND EDITION

Five years ago, I wrote a series of essays on gynecological diseases commonly encountered in American clinical practice. These essays were then bound together and published as *Free And Easy*. This book has sold consistently over the last five years, primarily to practitioners of Traditional Chinese Medicine (TCM), and now it is time to release a second edition. Every book has a life and this book's life is not yet spent. However, the state of the art for both myself and American TCM practitioners five years ago is hardly state of the art now. Therefore, I would like to take this opportunity to bring my readers up to date on the material contained herein. With these amendments, I hope this book will survive another five years before needing to be supplanted entirely.

The first essay on PMS, it seems to me, is still reasonably good. It does have, however, at least three short-comings. First, it over-emphasizes the role of the Liver in the disease mechanism of PMS. Although the Liver is, I still believe, the pivotal Organ in PMS, I did not say nearly enough about the Heart, Lungs, Stomach, and Large Intestine. Each of these Organs play an important role in some women's PMS to which I gave little or no attention. In part, this was due to my simplistic description of *Ke* cycle energetics. When the Liver invades

Earth, the Spleen does typically become Deficient and, over time, often Damp, but just as typically, the Stomach becomes Hot and Excess. This Stomach Heat *Xiang Sheng* or mutually arises with Liver Heat to accumulate in the Upper Burner disturbing the Heart and Lungs. This accounts for the weeping and emotional lability beyond just anger and depression. When one takes these other Organs into account, treatment strategies, both herbal and acupuncture, become more numerous, more individually comprehensive, and more effective.

Secondly, probably due to my own anger and frustration, I believe I over-emphasized these two emotions as the most important etiological factors in PMS. This also seems simplistic to me now. I think the pace at which we live, our diet, and typical lack of both adequate exercise and deep relaxation all play an important part in this and other Chinese Liver diseases beyond just pent up anger and frustration.

And third, my opinions about orthomolecular therapy and Western phytotherapy were neither informed nor particularly insightful. Orthomolecular therapy means the therapeutic use of vitamins, minerals, enzymes, co-enzymes, co-factors, and amino and fatty acids which occur in the human body and which are essential in the proper balance to maintain proper function. In the last year, I have begun using orthomolecular therapy quite successfully in adjunct to Chinese herbal medicine. This is based on my having worked out TCM descriptions of the basic vitamins, minerals, and amino acids, and some enzymes, co-enzymes, and fatty acids. Using such a combination of herbs and orthomolecular formulae, I now achieve quite good results in treating most women's PMS in 45 days instead of 90.

Western phytotherapy means the use of Western herbal ingredients medicinally. Five years ago I had not worked out the TCM descriptions of Evening Primrose Oil or Borage Oil, and, therefore, never used these medicinals in my PMS treatment plans even though I was well aware of their empirical efficacy. Now, I often use such Western herbal ingredients, because of their efficacy, easy administration, and cost-effectiveness. When I do use Western medicinals, it is *always* based on a TCM understanding of their properties, functions, and indications and contraindications. This preface is not the place to attempt to describe such individual medicinals. Suffice it to say, I do intend to publish a Western herbal, vitamin/mineral, and Western medicine *Ben Cao* at some point in the future. As I have written elsewhere, the essence of TCM is a conceptual methodology which can be applied to any medicinal substance or therapy from any culture or locale. My current therapeutic repertoire has become more universal and not so parochially Chinese. Yet, hopefully, the rigor of my TCM process has become even more precise and stringent.

In my vaginitis essay, I feel I also made three important mistakes. The first was a methodological mistake concerning the categorization of vaginitis as a disease in TCM. Following Jeremy Ross' lead, I discussed vaginitis under the TCM heading *Dai Xia* or abnormal vaginal discharge. Although vaginitis is often accompanied by *Dai Xia*, vaginitis, meaning inflammation and sores on the vagina, is discussed under the heading *Yin Shi* (erosion of genitalia) and *Re Chuang* (Hot lesions, i.e. herpes genitalia) within *Pi Fu Ke* or dermatology in Chinese medicine. *Fu Ke*, gynecology, is a subdivision of *Nei Ke* or Internal medicine. *Pi Fu Ke* is a subdivision of *Wai Ke* or External medicine. Therefore, vaginitis, a dermatological condition in Chinese medicine, is not discussed in *Fu Ke* texts. This emphasizes the point that Chinese medicine has its own logical divisions and categorizations different from Western medicine and that Western practitioners need to familiarize ourselves with these Chinese categorizations in order to know where in the Chinese literature to do our research. I myself was not clear about this until 1988 when I helped translate a Chinese clinical dermatology manual.

My second mistake was in hypothesizing both an External and an Internal etiology for herpes genitalia. My understanding of viral diseases has increased dramatically in the last five years, and I no longer think herpes can be generated entirely Internally. Rather, I would describe it as a *Fu Wen Xie*, a Hidden Warm Evil, which can remain latent until the Internal environment allows for the Evil's active flourishing. I have quite a bit more to say about such viral diseases in my soon to be released *Cervical Dysplasia & Prostate Cancer: HPV, The Hidden Link* which addresses this subject in detail.

The third important mistake in this essay was a wrong, superficial appraisal of the role of candida in vaginal infections, in particular, and in chronic disease, in general, and the efficacy of Western anti-candidiasis regimes. I have now come to see the importance of polysystemic chronic candidiasis (PSCC) in many of my patients' conditions and now treat candidiasis directly and deliberately. However, as a TCM practitioner, I could not do this conceptually until I identified candidiasis as a parasite (*Chong*) under the *Bu Nei Bu Wai Yin* (Neither Internal Nor External) category of disease causation. Once I was able to see candidiasis from that perspective, I have been able to utilize a much fuller, more comprehensive collection of therapies to address this condition more directly in my patients. This includes hypoallergenic, yeast -free meal replacements, candidicidal herbs and orthomolecular supplements, and bacteria replacement therapy. All these can be rationally prescribed based on a legitimate TCM diagnosis once one sees candidiasis as a parasite condition requiring the principle of *Sha Jun* or killing fungus. Treating candidiasis consciously and deliberately can help many patients who otherwise seem unusually complex, sensitive, or recalcitrant to Chinese herbal treatment alone. I also discuss the TCM treatment of candidiasis in greater detail in *Cervical Dysplasia & Prostate Cancer.*

In the cervical dysplasia essay, my main over-sight was my total lack of discussion of its viral and venereal etiology. It is currently believed that most cervical dysplasia is due to venereally transmitted, viral infection. A series of retroviruses called human papilloma viruses (HPV) are implicated , as well as possibly some synergistic activity between HPV and HSV II (the herpes genitalia virus). This suggests that cervical dysplasia is also due, in TCM, to a species of *Fu Wen Xie* or Hidden Warm Evil.

The treatment of cervical dysplasia has become one of my specialties, and I have a whole volume more to say about it in *Cervical Dysplasia & Prostate Cancer.* In that book, I discuss the whole concept of a *Wen Bing* or Warm disease, Hidden Evils, and their reverse evolution in venereal diseases. In addition, I present a much more comprehensive treatment plan using orthomolecular therapy, Western phytotherapy, and modern homeopathy in addition to Chinese herbs and acupuncture. However, although my current treatment of cervical dysplasia is much more sophisticated and insightful than that presented in this book, the bottom line is that we *can indeed* treat this condition with routine efficacy. And, based on five years further clinical experience, I have also found that TCM can, in most instances, reverse even carcinoma in situ.

The fact that this second preface is necessary is itself telling about TCM in the West. Practitioners such as myself have had a difficult time learning Chinese medicine in English. When I began its study in the late seventies, there were only a bare handful of books available, which were often contradictory and confusing if not downright erroneous. Most of those early books on Oriental medicine were Macrobiotic, written by George Ohsawa, Naburo Muramoto, and Michio Kushi. Then there was the Ilza Veith translation of the *Nei Jing*, OICS' presentation of Nguyen Van Nghi's work, and *Essentials*. On top of that, there were the oral teachings of various Chinese Tai Ji and Gong Fu teachers and those of J.R. Worsley whose students at that time were the most visible American practitioners of acupuncture.

Slowly, slowly over the last ten years, translations have appeared from mainland China teaching the contemporary Chinese style called Traditional Chinese Medicine. In the last decade, this style (TCM) has largely come to dominate the American Oriental medicine scene. This style is a very systematic and methodological one which, at least in Chinese, is very clear and straightforward. However, because of the continued paucity of translations and American schools' as yet refusing to bite the bullet of requiring all their students to study modern medical Chinese, the level of Westerners ability to understand and do TCM even at a professional entry level is still growing.

Looking back over the essays in *Free And Easy*, it is both gratifying and disturbing to see how far my own understanding and ability to think TCM has matured. It is gratifying in that there is a sense of real progress and maturation. However, it is disturbing in that so many of us in the past and perhaps still are playing a very serious game without a full deck of cards. This game is serious because it involves the life and well-being of other people who come to us entrusting us with their care. That is a big responsibility -- one which requires sincerity, dedication, and perseverance. Looking back five years ago, my insights into TCM seem pretty pedestrian and exhibit to me now only bare competence. And yet, at the time of their writing, they were published in our profession's best American journals.

Hopefully, the next five years will see a consolidation of rudimentary, professional TCM education in this country. We can only hope for more translations of basic TCM texts and also increasing rigor at our colleges, both in admissions and in curriculum. It is still as yet presumptuous to think that our current TCM is on a par with a current Chinese graduate's. In preparing this second edition of *Free And Easy*, I have hopefully rectified the most obvious and egregious errors of the first edition so that the information contained herein may be considered basic entry level TCM.

PREFACE
TO THE FIRST EDITION

When I first began practicing Chinese medicine, an inadvertently large proportion of my patients were women. Since the menstrual cycle is a good indicator of the female patient's systemic balance, and, since women suffer from a number of gynecological problems not experienced by men, I naturally focused a great deal of attention on the pathophysiology of women vis a vis their menstrual cycle. As I became more knowledgable about the menstrual cycle and the factors which influence it, I consciously made the decision, at first largely to minimize my personal levels of stress, to specialize in this branch of Traditional Chinese Medicine known as *Fu Ke*. Once this decision was made, it brought me even more experience in this area, which, in turn, demanded further literary research and contemplation.

At this point in time, it is my opinion that American female patients are not the same as Chinese female patients. Although traditional Chinese *Zheng* or patterns of disharmony are, in most cases, accurate descriptions of the possibilities of human pathophysiology, American women are more likely to suffer from certain combinations of *Zheng* and from certain disorders than their Asian sisters. These epidemiological differences are due to differences in lifestyle, diet, prior medical treatment, and varying levels of physical, emotional, mental, and spiritual stress. It is my belief and experience that the American practitioner of Traditional Chinese Medicine must consciously take these differences into account, perhaps not so much when diagnosing as when erecting treatment plans.

Over the last two years I have written a number of articles on various gynecological problems commonly encountered amongst American women. Several of these have been published in *The American Journal of Acupuncture* and *The Journal of the American College of Traditional Chinese Medicine*. Although some of these articles survey all the commonly accepted Chinese *Zheng* for each disorder, still, it is my experience that the majority of American women suffer from Liver Qi Congestion and a tendency towards Yin Deficiency. Therefore, because of the importance of the Liver in women's diseases in general and in American women in particular, I have entitled this collection of essays *Free and Easy*. This is my translation of *Xiao Yao*, the name of an important gynecological formula for dredging the Liver, benefitting the Spleen, and tonifying the Blood. Its name implies that the necessary corrective for Liver Qi Congestion is the development and maintenance of a free and easy attitude.

The development of a free and easy attitude and thus a free and unobstructed flow of Qi and Blood is no easy task for late twentieth century Americans. And I think it is even more difficult for women than men because of their uncertain role and position in our society. Consequently, I believe that the American practitioner must pay more attention to their female patients' diet, lifestyle, exercise, and emotional well-being than the average practitioner in China. In my experience, in China, typically the clincan will offer only a few simple suggestions, such as "Don't worry". Although such counsel is no less germane here, such simple advice is too often simplistic. American stress is so pervasive that I have *never* felt an

American patient's pulse completely lose its wiry quality. Although Chinese herbal medicine and acupuncture can usually alleviate the symptoms of Liver Qi Congestion and Yin Deficiency, they can seldom eradicate these particular patterns in the young American urban adult.

On the one hand, this is a bit depressing. On the other, it should force the American clinician to look deeper into the causes of these patterns of imbalance amongst so many Americans. Zhu Dan-xi, in *Dan Xi Xin Fa Hu Dan*, states that psychological conflicts causing energetic imbalance must be resolved *on their own level*. Since, in my opinion, most gynecological problems amongst American women are caused or aggravated by our society's pervasive and unrelieved stress, treatment plans for their rebalancing must address these issues. Once having a clearer understanding of the depth and extent of the cultural, sociological, dietary, and iatrogenic etiologies of these patterns, hopefully we as clinicians can help our patients to erect treatment plans that encompass more than just professionally prescribed herbal medicine or professionally administered acupuncture. Should this be the case, then the American practice of Chinese medicine will truly embody a profound, preventive, and holistic approach to human healthcare.

At the least, I hope that the inclusion of previously untranslated material from Chinese gynecological texts and case histories will enable American practitioners to diagnose and treat their American women patients more accurately and effectively. I believe gynecology, in particular, is one of the specialties of Traditional Chinese Medicine which, both in terms of theory and effective treatment, compares more than favorably with the Western allopathic approach. Chinese gynecological pathophysiology contains a wisdom which can enable the practitioner to truly treat preventively. In addition, its treatment modalities are all low in iatrogenic impact and free of side-effects if accurately chosen and correctly administered. Therefore, in advancing the knowledge of traditional Chinese gynecology in American, I hope these essays, in some small way, contribute to the alleviation of pain and suffering in those who hold up half the sky.

TABLE OF CONTENTS

PREMENSTRUAL SYNDROME (PMS)

In the last several years numerous articles have appeared in scholarly journals and in popular magazines describing Premenstrual Syndrome or PMS. The appearance of these articles make it seem like there is a PMS epidemic among American women in their twenties and thirties. As an American practitioner of Traditional Chinese Medicine specializing in gynecology it sometimes seems that way to me too. In the last few years I have had quite a bit of experience in treating PMS and I believe Chinese medicine offers the best explanations for this syndrome, both individually and epidemiologically, as well as the most effective treatment plans. As Ted Kaptchuk points out in *The Web That Has No Weaver,* a syndrome from the Western point of view means a group of signs and symptoms which typically occur together for which as yet there is no satisfactory explanation.[1] Chinese medicine, however, not only recognizes the symptoms of the syndrome as a pattern, but does in fact define the etiology of this pattern.

Before we present the energetic imbalance which is the cause of Premenstrual Syndrome, we must first outline the main symptoms of this problem. The single most important symptom is emotional lability preceding the onset of menstruation each month. Emotional lability is the opposite of emotional stability. It is commonly known as moodiness. Typically the most common and problematic emotions experienced by sufferers of PMS are depression, frustration, anger and irritability. These may be experienced for only a day or two each month directly preceding one's period or may last for several weeks each cycle in severe cases. Some women experience such deep depression each month they contemplate suicide and fear for their sanity. Not only is this emotional lability painful for the sufferer of PMS, but it also causes pain to family members and friends.

Other symptoms of PMS are cravings (especially for sweets), water retention, fatigue, diarrhea and/or constipation, the recurrent catching of a cold each month during the premenstrual period, abdominal bloating, breast swelling, tenderness and/or the presence of lumps, headaches, often including migraines, insomnia, sore throat, nausea, menstrual irregularity, and dysmenorrhea. Each and every one of these symptoms is explained by Chinese medical theory and is well treated by various combinations of traditional Chinese therapies.

The basic energetic imbalance which causes Premenstrual Syndrome according to Traditional Chinese Medicine is Liver Qi Congestion. In Chinese medicine the Liver is responsible for "spreading the Qi" and maintaining its smooth and unobstructed flow. This is called in the literature the patency of the Qi. This smooth and unobstructed flow implies that the right energy arrives at the right place at the right time. Energy or Qi in Chinese medicine means function. Therefore the cyclic flow of the Qi describes from the Chinese point of view the endocrine system and the rise and fall of hormones in the body. In Chinese medicine anything which harms the Liver may cause an obstruction in the flow of Qi in the body at large. Likewise, anything which obstructs the flow of Qi may also harm the Liver.

Liver Qi Congestion in females usually manifests as obstruction

2

in the flow of Qi in one of three areas of the body. The first
is in the pelvis. Although the classical Chinese knew the
physical liver is located below the ribs on the right side, they
relegated the Liver's function primarily to the lower abdomen.
The Liver is sometimes referred to as the *Xue Shi* or Blood
Chamber, which is also an appellation for the Uterus.[2]
Congestion in the Liver can cause congestion and stagnation of
Qi in the lower abdomen. This may result in flatulence, lower
abdominal bloating, menstrual irregularity, and dysmenorrhea.
The Qi moves the Blood. When the Qi becomes stuck, the
Blood may also stagnate. This, over a period of time, can lead
to the formation of neoplasms in the pelvis such as myomas,
fibromas, and ovarian cysts as well as to endometriosis and
chronic pelvis inflammatory disease.   In such cases the
menstrual discharge is usually dark and clotted.

The Penetrating Vessel (*Chong Mai*), the meridian or energy
pathway which runs up the core of the body, is also known as
the Sea of Blood. This likewise is an alternative name for the
Liver itself. When there is Liver Qi Congestion in the Lower
Burner or lower abdomen, this meridian is also affected. This
channel is intimately related to the reproductive organs and
cycle. When there is menstrual irregularity and dysmenorrhea,
it is always involved.[3]

The second area of the body that can manifest symptoms of
energy stagnation when the Liver Qi is congested is the chest.
This may manifest as a sensation of tightness or pressure in the
chest or below the diaphragm, but in women more often
presents as breast swelling, pain, and lumpiness. Frequent
sighing is one diagnostic sign of Liver Qi Congestion and these
sighs unconsciously seek to relieve this thoracic congestion.
The *Chong Mai* which arises from the Lower Burner and ends
in the chest, is usually involved when there is Liver Qi
Congestion manifesting in the chest or breasts.   This
Extraordinary meridian is also very important in relation to

3

menstruation and is linked to the Conception Vessel, both of which share a common source. In fact, in Chinese medical theory the two diagnostic patterns which pertain to disharmonies in these meridians imply that they become disordered together.[4]

Liver Qi Congestion can also manifest as stagnation in the area of the throat. This can range from neurotic esophageal stenosis or stricture, called in Chinese Plum Seed Qi, to hypertrophy of the thyroid gland and goiter.[5] Thyroid imbalance according to Western medicine can derange metabolic rate and subsequent maintenance of a steady weight and body temperature. Although frequent sore throats can be related to Liver Qi Congestion at the level of the throat, most typically the patient suffers from constriction of the throat or the sensation of something being stuck in the throat.

When the Liver Qi becomes congested it can have secondary effects on other Organs. Liver Qi Congestion is an Excess of energy in the Liver. According to Five Element theory, such as Excess is most likely to be vented on the Spleen. In this case, it is said that the Liver invades the Spleen. This deranges Spleen function. In Chinese medicine the Spleen stands for the entire process of digestion. If the Liver becomes Excess the Spleen will become Deficient. Spleen Deficiency can manifest as diarrhea and loose stools if the Spleen's transformative function is primarily affected or as constipation if the Spleen's transportive function is affected. In some cases both transformation and transportation are affected in which case there will be alternating constipation and loose stools. Since the flavor which tonifies the Spleen is Sweet, patients with Spleen Deficiency will often crave sweets. Unfortunately too much or too concentrated Sweet will only further weaken the Spleen.

4

The Spleen is also in charge of transformation and transportation of Water in the Body. If these functions are impaired there may be water retention either in the body tissue such as in facial edema and swelling of the hands and feet or Stagnation of Water in the Stomach. The accumulation of Water is a local Excess imposed upon a Spleen Deficiency. Such an accumulation of Water or Dampness is usually involved in any nausea that may be experienced in the premenstrual period and is usually involved in any migrainous headaches accompanied by vomiting.

The Spleen is also responsible for the creation of the Postnatal Qi out of the essence of ingested food and the creation of Blood from the *Jing* Essence plus Liquid. When the Spleen becomes weak due to an overbearing Liver, insufficient Qi is created which leads to fatigue and insufficient Blood is created which leads to anemia, insomnia, migraine headaches, and a generally Deficient constitution. Over a long period of time or if the Kidneys are inherently weak, further weakening of the Kidneys may occur since the Spleen Qi or Yang is ultimately derived from the Kidney Yang. In such cases there will be polyuria, nocturia, chronic cystitis, low back pain, weak knees, etc.

Because Qi is Yang, when the Liver Qi is congested or Excess, this Excess tends to transform into Heat and to flow up. Since the Liver is a Yin Organ it does not hold on to Yang energy. Instead it passes this Yang energy to its paired Yang Bowel, the Gallbladder. This Yang Qi flows up the Gallbladder meridian and is responsible for one-sided headaches and shoulder and neck tension.

The Liver stores the *Hun*. In classical Chinese medicine each of the Five *Zang* or solid Yin Organs is associated with a psycho-spiritual energy. The *Hun* is the psyche. When the Liver becomes congested, the *Hun* becomes agitated just as the

Shen which resides in the Heart becomes agitated when there is too much Heat in that Organ. This leads to Liver Qi Congestion insomnia which is to be distinguished from Heart Blood Deficiency insomnia and Stagnant Food insomnia.[6] It is also the cause of the emotional lability.

All the above scenarios can be attributed in one way or another to Liver Qi Congestion. Women who suffer from PMS always have some element of Liver Qi Congestion. Most typically the diagnosis also includes imbalance of the *Chong* and *Ren* channels and Spleen Deficiency, Blood Deficiency, and possible breakdown of the Spleen's ability to transform and transport Water. Each patient must be assessed as to the relative severity of each of the components in the diagnosis. Some women have more or less digestive difficulties. Others have more or less water retention. Others have more or less breast swelling, headaches, or depression. However, each of the major signs and symptoms associated with Premenstrual Syndrome can be accounted for by one or more of the above Chinese medical theories.

We could, at this point, go directly to a discussion of the treatment of this syndrome. However, before the treatment plan which I suggest will make sense, we must further discuss why this problem is so prevalent among modern women today.

According the Chinese medicine the Liver is the "temperamental" organ.[7] That means it is easily harmed by emotional upset. Specifically the Liver is most susceptible to the harmful effects of anger. Anger makes the Qi rise up rebelliously. Part of the mechanism of menstruation is a descension of Yang energy into the pelvis to mobilize the Blood for discharge. It is the failure of this energy to descend which causes the symptoms of Qi Stagnation whether at the throat, thorax, or lower abdomen. Premenstrual Syndrome is therefore, in my opinion, most significantly due to emotional factors. Most women with PMS report a more than average amount of emotional stress in their lives stretching back at least to puberty. Sometimes this upsetment is historical, but often the patient's life continues to be emotionally stressful.

To the idiosyncratic emotional history of the individual must also be added the generalized level of stress and upsetment endemic to our culture. Women's roles are in flux. Old role models have been rejected and new models may be emotionally unrealistic. Often modern women feel they should be superwomen. Many women who are single parents or career women try to manifest both traditional female roles of mother, homemaker, etc., with the masculine roles of breadwinner and business person. Stress is frustration. It is trying to do too much in a given period of time with inadequate resources. On an energetic level, frustration is an unfluid or impeded flow of Qi. Frustration also is an inherently aggressive or angry emotional state of trying to "push the river".

Not only is women's current role in society inherently stressful, but our entire lifestyle generates more stress that I believe the human organism is capable of withstanding without deleterious effect. Background noise from appliances like this computer, background music (especially rock 'n roll and discordant jazz), television, national and world news, driving in cars, pollution, denatured food, politics, the threat of nuclear war, the breakdown in the family, both nuclear and extended, the rise of terrifying diseases such as cancer, AIDS, etc., all cause us more stress than most of us are aware. In my practice I have come to expect red papillae on the tip of the tongue as standard. However, classically they are a sign of Heat building in the nervous system, i.e. the Liver and Heart according to Chinese medicine, due to stress. We have become accustomed to our abnormally high level of ambient stress without having accommodated to it. All this stress adds to any given woman's personal emotional turmoil.

7

As mentioned before, the Liver is responsible for the patency of Qi flow in the organism. This is equivalent to the Liver's governing and being effected by periodicity in general. Birth control pills, by adding to the system hormones out of phase with the body's normal periodicity, adversely affect the Liver's "spreading" function or the smooth and regular flow of Qi. This is why birth control pills are implicated in a higher than normal incidence of pelvic and breast neoplasms, both of which according to Chinese medicine begin as stuck Liver Qi. This is compounded by our culture's disregard for the periodicity of nature in our lifestyle. Women who are flight attendants have, in my experience, the most pronounced cases of Liver Qi caused imbalances. They are only the extreme end of our culture's disregard for the effect of astrology and geomancy on our systems. Chinese medicine stresses above all else the regular cyclic flow and periodicity of our internal energy which must remain in harmony with the larger rhythms of the universe, or what is called in classical Chinese Heaven. Both the use of birth control pills and inattention to natural periodicity in general are contributing factors in the cause of PMS.

Likewise, because the Liver is so intimately related to the Uterus and controls the circulation of the pelvis or Lower Burner, anything which harms either the tone or circulation of the Lower Burner will adversely affect the Liver Qi. Such things as abortions, IUDs, tubal ligations, appendectomies, and the suppression of infections in the Lower Burner by antibiotics all tend to weaken and impair the circulation of the Qi and Blood in the pelvis. If, due to trauma, such as caused by surgery or abortion, Stagnant Blood is created in the pelvis, this will eventually cause mental/emotional problems since the Qi and Blood mutually control one another and flow together. The flow of Qi is synonymous with the flow of emotions and anything which causes Stagnant Blood will cause Stagnant Qi and vice versa. Therefore the stress of abortions and surgery

8

are also contributing factors in this syndrome.

Finally, modern women's increasingly common decision to postpone or forego childbearing contributes to Liver Qi Congestion. Each month the menstrual discharge purges Evil Heat from the Blood. This Heat both comes from the Liver and affects the Liver. Likewise, when a woman has a baby the postpartum discharge or lochia is a similar discharge of *Xie Qi* on a much larger scale. In my book *Path Of Pregnancy* I discuss in greater detail the importance and management of this postpartum discharge. Women who do not have this discharge or who postpone it until later in life do not reap its benefits. Due to the decongesting effect possible from this discharge, many women experience a cessation of premenstrual problems after giving birth, i.e. their Liver Qi was discharged with their lochia. Also suckling, which promotes local flow in the breast, helps to relieve any tendency for stuck Qi to accumulate in that area and that is why breast feeding is associated with a lower incidence of breast cancer.

To recapitulate, I believe emotional stress and our society's unnatural lifestyle are to blame for the current epidemic of PMS among contemporary American women in their twenties and thirties. It is not just that someone has identified a problem which previously was not labeled and therefore never discussed. I believe there are ample reasons which suggest the rise in the incidence of this problem is real. That being the case, how can this problem be treated?

First, in terms of prevention I recommend avoiding the use of birth control pills and IUDs, avoiding surgery and antibiotics if at all possible, and minimizing stress as much as possible in one's daily life. I also recommend eating fresh natural foods, living with the natural macrocosmic rhythms, living among a support group of close friends if not family members, giving birth naturally, breast feeding, and having some spiritual

9

purpose to one's life which helps minimize existential anxiety, frustration, and irresponsibility.

For women who already have PMS, I must first counsel them on the importance of diet. Diet is not the primary cause of PMS. Diet alone I do not believe is a comprehensive treatment of PMS. But diet is an important adjunct to successful treatment. First it is most important to avoid foods which will tend to aggravate the Liver. These are alcohol, coffee, heavy red meats in excess, grease, oil, fatty, and fried foods, Spicy, Hot Pungent foods, overeating in general, eating heavy, hard-to-digest foods, and eating preservatives, chemicals, pollutants, and drugs, recreational, over-the-counter, or prescription, all of which must be detoxified by the Liver. In my experience, avoidance of as many of these as much as possible will by itself eliminate a certain percentage of the symptoms and severity of PMS.

I do not believe there are any foods which significantly alleviate Liver Qi Congestion. However, in women whose PMS is complicated by Spleen Deficiency or Water Stagnation there are foods which can be eaten which will be of benefit. These are cooked, warm, nourishing vegetables, chicken and beef broth, well-cooked and easily digestible grains in small amounts, and a cautious use of warming spices such as ginger, cardamom, cinnamon, nutmeg, etc. In cases of Spleen Deficiency with Dampness, cold and raw foods should be avoided, including raw fruits and vegetables. It is especially important not to drink cold liquids or any liquids in too large a quantity, not to eat ice cream or chilled foods, and if there is a production of mucous, not to eat milk and milk products.

As stated above, diet alone is not a sufficient treatment of PMS. But the more the symptomology of PMS involves digestive and Spleen-related imbalance, the more important is diet in the overall treatment plan. For those whose discomfort is mostly mental/emotional, diet is not as important. However, in all sufferers of PMS, the elimination of coffee from the diet is of utmost importance. This should be accomplished over a period of time in which the patient gradually diminishes her coffee consumption. Coffee us a very powerful herb or drug with profound effects on the Liver. The craving or use of coffee by PMS sufferers in understandable since it does give a temporary relief from the energy congestion. However, its net effect is to imbalance the Liver even further. The practitioner should be aware that the craving for coffee is an addiction and the patient should be helped to deal with that addiction in any way appropriate. Some Chinese practitioners suggest the application of a few drops of *White Flower Oil* on the tip of the tongue whenever the patient feels the need for a cup of coffee. This peppermint-based oil will decongest the Liver Qi and therefore provide the feeling of a "burst" of energy which will not harm the Liver but on the contrary actually be of some benefit. For further information on the rationale and treatment plan for treating Liver Qi Congestion, the reader should see my book on Chinese dietary therapy, *Prince Wen Hui's Cook.*

The second therapy I suggest to patients with Premenstrual Syndrome is exercise. When we sit, the Blood in our arms and legs returns to the Liver for storage. This pooling of Blood in the Liver tends to aggravate Liver Qi Congestion. Exercise pumps this Blood out of the Liver and along with it some of the stuck Qi. Also, according to the Five Element theory, the Lungs control the Liver and keep it from becoming Excess. Exercise which strengthens the Lungs can help keep the Liver under control. For exercise to be a significant therapy for Liver Qi Congestion it must be aerobic in nature. That means that although walking is healthful, one must raise her heart rate and respiration to almost double and keep it at that level for a minimum of twenty minutes. No significant further benefit is derived from such exercise after thirty minutes in terms of treating the Liver Qi and it need not be done every day. Every other day or every seventy-two hours is sufficient. Aerobics classes, dancercise, swimming, running, racquetball, basketball, all can be aerobic exercise. However, it is my opinion that although exercise is of great benefit and importance in treating stuck Liver Qi, it only bleeds off the Excess as if venting steam from a pressure cooker. It does not remedy the production of the Excess at its root.

What will get at the root of the production of Excess Qi stagnating in the Liver is deep relaxation. This is the third therapy I always prescribe in such cases. And, although I present it third, I stress its preeminence in the treatment plan. Deep relaxation, I believe, more than anything else remedies the effects of stress and emotional upset. I believe, in fact, deep relaxation alone without counselling or psychotherapy is sufficient to heal most psychoemotional problems. However, in order for deep relaxation to be therapeutically effective, certain criteria must be met.

First, it must include the whole body; it must be muscular relaxation, not just cerebral relaxation. Second, it must result in the center of consciousness to come out of the head and reside below the level of the navel in what is called by the Chinese the Lower *Tan Tian*. Third, it must be done for a minimum of twenty minutes per day but does not need to be done for more than thirty minutes. And fourth, it must be done every day without missing a single day for at least the first one hundred days.

Although there are a number of techniques to accomplish this kind of deep relaxation available, such as meditation, hatha yoga and biofeedback, I believe the most efficient is the daily use of a relaxation tape. There are many types of meditation, many of which do not relax the physical body nor lower the center of consciousness "below the belt". This relaxation is being prescribed therapeutically and not for primarily spiritual reasons. Ven. Trogawa Rinpoche, a famous Tibetan Lama Doctor who is equally a teacher of the Dharma, prescribes such deep relaxation even to Buddhist meditators on top of their daily meditation since the two endeavors do not necessarily achieve the same result. Biofeedback is excellent but it is expensive. And hatha yoga may be more time-consuming than what can be done every single day. Relaxation tapes are cheap and require relatively little discipline. They are usually made in such a way as to include subliminal commands to relax imbedded in their pacing, tone, background noise or music, and phrasing. The time of day one does this relaxation is not crucial, only that the patient establishes a regular time every day to "do" the tape.

Although this is the single most effective thing the patient can do for herself, I introduce it last among these Three Free Therapies since many patients have resistance to this type of therapy, discount its effectiveness, or assume they are relaxed. If this is the case, I allow patients to first implement the first two therapies, diet and exercise, while continuing to counsel gently for the introduction of this third. Those of my patients who have been willing and faithful in doing this deep relaxation have always had good results.

Next we come to the main professionally administered therapies for PMS according to Chinese medicine. They are internal herbal treatment and acupuncture. In my practice I favor the use of herbs in the treatment of chronic problems since they are time and cost effective for the patient, are taken three times a day so their stimulus is fairly constant, and also since they work from the inside out on a chemical or cellular level. In my experience, using Chinese herbal formulae one can eliminate over 50% of all PMS symptoms in three menstrual cycles. In many cases one can eliminate all symptoms of PMS within that same period. Initially I use custom-blended bulk herbs in substantial doses, i.e. from 3 to 12 grams per day per ingredient in decoction. Once improvement has been made I often switch my patients to a powdered extract of the same formula at a much lower dose, one to three grams per day per ingredient, or to a Chinese proprietary medicine in pill form. These two methods are even more cost effective and time efficient for the patient and lend themselves to the consolidation of therapeutic effect after the major symptomology has been relieved. In treating Premenstrual Syndrome with Chinese herbs, attention must be paid to timing, some times in the cycle requiring a stronger dose or the inclusion of certain ingredients not necessary at other times in the cycle.

Chinese herbal formulae must be prescribed on the basis of Traditional Chinese Medical diagnosis. Therefore, before examining the basic formula for the treatment of this problem and its variation, we must first review the various Chinese patterns on which these variations are based. Liver Qi Congestion without Spleen Deficiency will manifest as depression, irritability, tension headaches, lower abdominal bloating, hypochondral or intercostal pain and soreness, a wiry pulse, and a normal or somewhat darkish, brownish tongue. There will tend to be menstrual irregularity and cramping, swelling of the breasts, and frequent sighing. There may also be constipation or variability of the color of the stools. Liver Qi Congestion with Spleen Deficiency manifests as loose stools, cold hands and feet, fatigue, pallor, a craving for sweets and/or a lack of appetite, indigestion, a pale tongue, possibly enlarged, and a wiry, deep, and slowish or relaxed pulse. Liver Qi Congestion with Damp Spleen manifests as constipation alternating with loose stools, sluggishness, a heavy feeling in the body, a fluted, swollen tongue, and a slippery, wiry pulse. If there is Stagnant Water, there may be a sloshing sound of liquid in the Stomach, water retention, thirst and a craving for water *which should not be indulged*, and incomplete urination.

The tongue may look moist and the pulse may feel fine and soggy. If there is Blood Deficiency complicating the case, the tongue will be pale and the pulse thready and fine. If there is Blood Stagnation, the pulse may be astringent, deep, or hesitant and the tongue purplish, brownish, or have ecchymotic patches along its edges. These patterns are only approximate, and often in clinical practice one meets with patients whose tongue or pulse does not meet one's textbook expectations. If, however, the practitioner is astute, he or she should be able to account theoretically for any unusual variations in the pulse or tongue.

The above are the major Chinese patterns of disharmony responsible for PMS. In sufferers of Premenstrual Syndrome, they are all variations of a basic Liver Qi Congestion. That syndrome is, in my experience, the key to this problem. Since the majority of American women with PMS are a combination of Liver Excess and Spleen Deficiency, the basic Chinese herbal formula I employ most often is called Xiao Yao San. This translates as Free and Easy Powder. The term "Free and Easy" is met with in the *Inner Chapters* of Chuang Tzu.[9] The name of this formula has also been translated as Leisure Powder by the editors of the *Journal of the American College of Traditional Chinese Medicine,* and as Bupleurum and Peony Combination in all books and periodicals published by the Oriental Healing Arts Institute. In *Commonly Used Chinese Herb Formulas With Illustrations,* it is listed as a Harmonizing formula, in this case harmonizing the Liver and the Spleen and the Conception Vessel and the *Chong Mai.*[10] Its ingredients are:

Radix Bupleuri
Radix Paeoniae Albae
Radix Angelicae Sinensis
Sclerotium Poria Cocoris
Rhizoma Atractylodis Albae

15

Radix Praeparata Glycyrrhizae
Rhizoma Recens Zingiberis

Bupleurum, Peony, and Dang Gui "soften" and "dredge" the Liver and regulate the *Chong* and *Ren Mai*. Poria, Atractylodes, Licorice, and Ginger tonify the Spleen and improve digestion. Peony and Dang Gui tonify the Blood; while Poria and Atractylodes tonify the Qi. Licorice and Ginger help to promote circulation.

Depending on the case, additions and deletions are made to this basic formula in order to tailor it to the individual. If Liver Qi Congestion is transforming into Fire due to Liu Wansu's Law of Similar Transformation, Cortex Radicis Moutan and Fructus Gardeniae are added to clear the Liver of Heat and cool the Blood. In such cases there will be a rapid pulse, a red tongue, and a bitter taste in the mouth upon arising in the morning. Such patients often have insomnia, excessive or violent dreams, irascibility, more serious depression, and migraines. If there is insomnia due to Ascension of Yang, also add Os Draconis and Concha Ostreae and have the patient take 1 gram of powdered Succinum one hour before retiring.

If there is Spleen Qi Deficiency, add more Poria and Atractylodes. Radix Astragali Seu Hedysari can also be added to tonify the Qi. This is especially useful if these are night sweats due to Blood Deficiency. For Blood Deficiency also add Radix Ligustici Wallichi and Radix Rehmanniae Conquitae to the formula. If there is a Dampness in the Spleen manifesting as loose stools and a moist white tongue fur, reduce the relative amounts of Peony and Dang Gui and add Rhizoma Pinelliae and Fructus Amomi Cardamomi. In cases which involve Stagnant Water and edema, add Rhizoma Alismatis, Semen Plantaginis, Semen Phaseoli, and Stigma Zeae Mays. For breast distention add Semen Citri and the two types of Pericarpium Citri Reticulatae (*Chen Pi & Qing Pi*). For

Yin Deficiency with a dry, red tongue, and lack of fur, delete Bupleurum and Ginger and add Fructus Ligustri Lucidi. For dysmenorrhea add Rhizoma Corydalis, Rhizoma Cyperi, and Radix Saussureae Seu Vladimiriae. On the day of the pain also add a small amount of Myrrha. For Stagnant Blood add Radix Salviae Miltorrhizae, Semen Persicae, Pericarpium Citri Reticulatae, and Herba Artemesiae Capillaris.[11] For Dry Intestine constipation add Pericarpium Citri Reticulatae Viride and Radix Trichosanthis. For migraines one must assess the relative proportions of Liver Qi Congestion, Water Stagnation, and Blood Deficiency. However, consider the addition of the Dang Gui tails, Radix Paeoniae Rubrae, Spica Prunellae, Semen Cassiae Torae, and Semen Sinapis Albae.

As one can see, this formula can be modified to fit the great majority of symptoms which manifest as Premenstrual Syndrome. The formula should be administered as soon as the symptoms of PMS begin to appear and it should be continued up through the first day of the period. During the rest of the month the formula should be taken either as powdered extract or as a patent pill. The extract available from Qualiherbs in Santa Fe Springs, CA as Bupleurum and Peony Combination includes Cortex Radicis Moutan and Fructus Gardeniae. So do the patent pills made by the Min-kang Drug Manufactory. Those made by the Lanchow Chinese Medicine Works only include the basic Free and Easy Powder formula. After significant results have been achieved the patient should continue to take the pills or powder for several months to consolidate the therapeutic effect. During times of stress or at the first sign of a relapse, the patient should be advised to resume medication. Since this problem is to some extent a personality disorder one will have a tendency to fall back into this pattern.

Other herbal formulae may, in certain cases, prove to be more appropriate than Free and Easy Powder, although Xiao Yao

San is the most common formula I prescribe to women with PMS. If there is emotional lability, constriction of the throat, suppressed anger and resentment, and Water Stagnation in the abdomen, the Decoction of Four and Seven is indicated. Minor Bupleurum Combination is indicated in women who catch cold before each period. However, I find it advisable to supplement this with Four Ingredient Decoction to tonify the Blood simultaneously. Women who experience chronic appendicitis or irritable bowel syndrome should use Bupleurum and Cinnamon Combination as the basis of their treatment with additions and deletions. If there is more pronounced breast involvement to the point of fibrocystic disease, Dang Gui Sixteen Herb Combination is suggested. In any case, one should not simply prescribe Free and Easy Powder on the basis of the Western diagnosis of Premenstrual Syndrome.

Although I prefer to use Chinese herbal formulae as the basis in my treatment of PMS, acupuncture can and does play a part. Generally I suggest an acupuncture treatment every other day or three times per week beginning at the onset of premenstrual symptoms. The major points which I use are Liver 3 (*Tai Chong*), and Large Intestine 4 (*He Gu*), the so-called Four Gates, to open up the flow of Qi throughout the entire body. To these I usually add Spleen 6 (*San Yin Jiao*) and Pericardium 6 (*Nei Guan*). Spleen 6 regulates the menstruation, promotes the flow of Qi in the pelvis, and relaxes the Liver. Pericardium 6 harmonizes the Liver and Spleen, improves circulation of Qi in the chest, and calms the Spirit. Depending on the other symptoms other points can be added to these. For instance: Bladder 20 (*Pi Shu*) and Stomach 36 (*Zu San Li*) for Spleen Deficiency; Conception Vessel 12 (*Zhong Wan*) and 9 (*Shui Fen*) and Spleen 9 (*Yin Ling Quan*) for Water Stagnation; Gallbladder 34 (*Yang Ling Quan*), Kidney 6 (*Zhao Hai*), Triple Heater 6 (*Zhi Gou*) and Stomach 25 (*Tian Shu*) for constipation; and Spleen 10 (*Xue Hai*), Conception Vessel 4 and 6 (*Guan Yuan & Qi Hai*),

Bladder 25 (*Da Chang Shu*), and Stomach 29 (*Gui Lai*) for Blood Stagnation dysmenorrhea, etc. There are many different styles of acupuncture and combinations to achieve similar results. Some acupuncturists prefer to use the Yang meridians; others prefer to use the Yin. Some acupuncturists tend to use a very limited repertoire of the most major points; others like to use less commonly used points such a Spleen 5 (*Shang Qiu*) for Spleen Dampness. The important thing is to discriminate the Root and Branch and to treat each accordingly. Care must always be taken to regulate the digestion since the Middle Burner is the source of Qi and Blood. Likewise, digestion cannot take place efficiently if the Stomach is full of water.

Acupuncture quickly relieves the symptoms of depression and bloating. Usually women getting up from the table notice immediate relief from sore and swollen breasts and swollen abdomen. I prefer to use acupuncture as a problem-solving, short-term therapy, to use a term borrowed from psychotherapy. Generally my PMS patients only require acupuncture the first couple of months of treatment and it is always given during the premenstrual period. If a woman's PMS began at ovulation the first month of therapy, I expect her PMS and the need for acupuncture will not manifest until one week before menstruation the second month of therapy. One sign that the treatment is headed in the right direction is a healthier looking menstrual discharge with brighter, fresher, less clotty blood which is neither too copious nor too scant. This is a good sign that the acupuncture and the herbs have had a beneficial effect and that not as much acupuncture will be needed in the future. However, the first discharge after beginning therapy may be clotty which may be a good sign that any Stagnant Blood is being expelled. In such a case one has to wait until the next discharge before making any firm conclusions.

There is one important point which should be mentioned

concerning the administration of acupuncture to Liver Qi Congested patients. These patients are invariably angry. They may not express this consciously or overtly but often vent their resentment and hostility unconsciously or covertly. They will often complain about the acupuncture and the difficulty of following their therapy. In their questions and answers they often unconsciously try to prove the therapist is wrong or mistaken. This is only a symptom of an "Angry Liver" and the practitioner should strive to remain centered and not become upset by this. In some cases, should the patient become angry during the treatment, this itself is a sign that the treatment has been effective in discharging anger from the Liver.

Some patients report that they feel disconnected or "spaced out" after receiving acupuncture for Liver Qi Congestion. They may complain about this feeling and may be reluctant to receive any more acupuncture if they expect this same feeling again. It is possible that some patients may even feel disconnected after taking their herbal formula, although I have had only two women who complained of this. Since the treatment opens up the flow of Qi and releases the energy which heretofore has been dammed up inside, it is natural for some women to experience this as a negative sensation. Really what these women are feeling is deep relaxation and freedom to which they are unaccustomed. Other patients who are not so "up tight" will experience these same sensations very positively. I have seen one patient who received acupuncture and herbal therapy for Liver Qi Congestion from a very reputable and well-educated Chinese doctor. She stopped therapy because she related to the sensations of freedom and ease as "losing her mind". She feared for her sanity since she could not "hold herself together anymore". Of course, this patient's excessive effort to hold herself and her world in a rigid pattern was the cause of her Congested Liver Qi. Because Liver Qi Congestion causes and is intimately associated with personality disorders, the practitioner who chooses to work with such patients must be prepared to deal with their emotional lability.

American patients will often ask about simultaneous taking of vitamin and mineral supplements and other remedies along with Chinese herbs. B vitamins, E, and minerals I believe are beneficial in the treatment of PMS. I think they are useful in alleviating the symptoms although I do not think they offer a radical cure. Vitamin C is counterproductive in PMS patients if, and most typically they are, suffering from Spleen Deficiency. Vitamin C is Cold energetically and can cause loose stools. Patients with Deficiency Cold or loose stools should not take mega doses of Vitamin C or it will further deplete their Righteous Qi. Many women ask about taking additional Dang Gui in capsule form. According to Chinese Medicine, the therapeutic dosage of Dang Gui is 4 to 9 grams per day. Most commercial Dang Gui is marketed in 500 mg. capsules which means that one would have to take 8 to 18 per day to receive any remarkable therapeutic effect. Also, in professional Chinese medicine, individual herbs are not used, but rather formulae. Dang Gui is an ingredient in most Chinese PMS related formulae, but by itself Dang Gui will not comprehensively relieve all the varying symptoms of Premenstrual Syndrome. It will only redress those symptoms related primarily to Blood Deficiency.

Other supplements such a Evening Primrose Oil are not described energetically by Traditional Chinese Medicine and therefore I can pass no judgment on them. The tendency in America to opt for shotgun therapy and to operate under the assumption that if a little is good more must be better are themselves indicative of a tight Liver always trying to push Mother Nature. Chinese medicine suggests that it is this very style of relating to reality which contributes to the development of PMS.

21

The following five case histories each exemplify a variation in the Chinese diagnosis and treatment of PMS. Each patient received the dietary, exercise and relaxation recommendations given above. They also each received Chinese herbal therapy and a selective use of acupuncture.

Case #1: A 30 year old woman complained of PMS for 2-1/2 years. It began when she started a new, more stressful job. Eight months after the onset of PMS she had an abortion after which all her symptoms got markedly worse. Her symptoms included insomnia, edema in her hands, feet, and face, swollen and painful breasts, stiff shoulders, anxiety, depression, and formication in her legs. Her tongue shape, color, and fur were all normal except for a pronounced red tip. Her pulse was thready and wiry. The patient also had very cold hands and feet and was easily chilled.

My diagnosis was Liver Qi Congestion, *Chong* and *Ren* imbalance, and Spleen Deficiency causing maltransportation and transformation of Water. I prescribed Free and Easy Powder in extract. She took 2 grams 3 times per day. Ten days before the expected date of her period she came for acupuncture. She mentioned that her stools were a little wet and loose. Her acupuncture treatment consisted of needling Stomach 36, Liver 3, Pericardium 6, Spleen 6, and moxaing Conception Vessel 12 and Bladder 20. Three days later she returned for her second treatment. Her stools had firmed up but she was very depressed. Her breasts were sore and her lower abdomen bloated. I needled Liver 3 and 5 (*Li Gou*), Pericardium 6, Spleen 6, and Conception Vessel 6 and moxaed Bladder 20. Two days later the patient was still anxious and depressed and still swollen. She received the same treatment as the previous one. Again two days later the patient was feeling much better. She was not swollen but now she was constipated. Her treatment on this day consisted of needling Stomach 25, Kidney 6, Triple Heater 6 (*Zhi Gou*), Gallbladder

34, Stomach 36, and Spleen 6, which rectified the constipation that day.

The patient stayed on Free and Easy Powder the next month. Two weeks before her period her breasts were swollen, she was still depressed, but she had no other symptoms. Her treatment consisted of needling Gallbladder 34, Stomach 34 (*Liang Qiu*), Liver 3, Spleen 6, Pericardium 6, and Conception Vessel 7 (*Yin Jiao*). She did not seek further acupuncture for ten days. On the fourth day before her period she reported that she was doing much better. Her sleep was much improved and there was no emotional lability. Her breasts were a little swollen and she was constipated. Her treatment was the same as the preceding one. Two days later the patient was no longer constipated but her breasts and eyes were still a bit swollen. On this day her acupuncture treatment consisted of needling the same formula minus Gallbladder 34.

The next month the patient accompanied me to China to study *Tuina* remedial massage at the Shanghai College of Traditional Chinese Medicine. While there we did our internship at the Yue Yang Hospital. The patient asked to see a Traditional Chinese doctor in the gynecology department. This gynecologist made exactly the same diagnosis and prescription. However, a number of Water-removing herbs were added to the formula, such as Semen Plantaginis, Corn Silk, Red Beans, etc., which were administered in decoction. In addition, she was given the basic Free and Easy formula in pill form to take on top of the decoction. She took the herbs in decoction and the pills for one month after which she continued only the patent medicine pills.

Three months later the patient received an acupuncture treatment for premenstrual bloating, depression, and water retention. Her treatment consisted of needling Spleen 6, Liver 5, Conception Vessel 6, Spleen 9, and Stomach 29. In the last six months the patient has not felt any further need for acupuncture and reports that her premenstrual discomfort is minimal. She is exceedingly grateful for the benefits of Traditional Chinese Medicine in dealing with this problem which was not only painful to her but also threatened her marriage. She continues to take Free and Easy formula in pill form to maintain and consolidate the therapeutic result.

Case #2: A 22 year old woman complained of extreme mood swings and uncontrolled depression and anger. She had been diagnosed as having PMS two years previously by a Western MD. One year before she had cyro-surgery to "remedy" cervical dysplasia. One month later she had a miscarriage. Two months after that she was diagnosed as having more dysplasia. Three months later she had PID for which she was given antibiotics. She developed a yeast infection subsequent to taking the antibiotics. Three months after that she developed cystitis, was again given antibiotics, and again developed a yeast infection. Another three weeks later she developed a yeast infection, cystitis, and a yeast infection in that order. The day before coming to see me and one month after the last round of infections, her boyfriend had been diagnosed as having non-specific urethritis.

This woman's menses had been regular but recently had become irregular, sometimes early, sometimes late. Her flow had become short, darker and more clotty after her first bout of dysplasia. She had "intolerable" dysmenorrhea on the first day of her period which caused diarrhea and nausea. She also had low back pain and "hot" pain in her thighs.

Other premenstrual symptoms included tensions headaches, pain and swelling in her breasts, water retention in her hands, thirst, a gain in body weight of 3 - 6 lbs., a ravenous craving for food and then a sudden loss of appetite and nausea, and bad sleep and nightmares for two weeks each month beginning at

24

ovulation. Her bowel movements were normal as was her urination. The patient drank coffee and had a problem with alcoholism. Her tongue color and shape were normal except for a red tip. The coating was a little thick and greasy to the rear. Her pulse was fast, fine, and wiry and sunken and weak bilaterally at the Foot position.

Her diagnosis was Liver Qi Congestion, Deficient Spleen *Qi Hua* function vis a vis Water metabolism, Damp Heat hidden in the Lower Burner, and Stagnant Blood in the Blood Chamber. Since the patient was immediately premenstrual at the time of diagnosis I prescribed the proprietary medicine Unborn Fawn Pills to decongest Stagnant Qi and Blood in the Lower Burner and Yili Analgesic Pills for relief of intense dysmenorrhea. During her period she had worse cramps than normal. The Analgesic Pills helped when she was finally able to take them. Her discharge was clottier and heavier but toward the end flowed a fresh, healthy red, which it had not done since the cyro-surgery. After her period I prescribed and the patient began taking Free and Easy Powder in extract form.

When her PMS began again eleven days before her period at approximately ovulation, the patient received acupuncture at Liver 3, Spleen 6, Stomach 36, Pericardium 6, Conception Vessel 4, and Stomach 29. Two days later she reported that she was having horrible mood swings, fluctuating from manic to suicidal. I altered her acupuncture to treat the Stagnant Blood since I felt that the Congested Qi liberated by the last treatment had simply "run headfirst" into the Stagnant Blood in her pelvis. Her treatment, therefore, consisted of needling Spleen 6 and 10, Liver 2 (*Xing Jian*), Conception Vessel 4, and Stomach 29. I also prescribed Free and Easy Decoction from bulk herbs at a heavy dosage (average 9 grams per ingredient) with the addition of Rhizoma Cyperi, Flos Carthami, and Semen Persicae. After this treatment the patient felt more

25

emotionally stable and calm. Two days later we repeated the same procedure. When her period came she had almost no cramping at all. Her discharge was longer and heavier but still dark.

The second full cycle after beginning treatment, this patient's PMS began one week before her period, not at ovulation as previously. She had continued to take the Free and Easy Powder in extract throughout the month. When she came in six days before her period we needled Liver 3, Spleen 6, 8 (*Di Ji*), and 10, Conception Vessel 4, Stomach 29. Pericardium 6, and Large Intestine 4. I gave her three *bao* or packets of Free and Easy Decoction, 1 *bao* equalling 2 days' dose. Safflower and Persica were added to the basic formula. The patient only felt she needed the one acupuncture treatment, which was considered a big improvement. Her period was almost pain-free. Her discomfort was limited to diffuse cramping as opposed to her previous stabbing pain. This indicated the Stagnant Blood was much better. To corroborate this, her discharge was a fresh, bright red.

The following month this patient came in one time one week before her period. Although she had been under a lot of stress and she had expected a relapse, her mental depression and irritability were comparatively slight. Her major complaint was breast swelling and nipple tenderness. She had taken Free and Easy Powder, again in extract form, all month and again I supplied her with 3 *bao* of bulk herbs to last for 6 days. I added Rhizoma Cordyalis, Radix Sausurreae Seu Vladimiriae, Rhizoma Cyperi, and both types of Pericarpium Citri Reticulatae. She received acupuncture at Liver 3, Pericardium 6, Large Intestine 4, Spleen 6, Conception Vessel 4, and Stomach 34. Her breast soreness was immediately diminished as soon as she got up off the table. She did not seek further treatment that cycle and her period was once again much less painful and the Blood was fresher and brighter.

26

Although this woman's therapy is not complete, as of this writing, she has shown gratifying results in the short space of three months. Her mental symptoms were the worst that I have encountered in a PMS patient. My prognosis for this patient is optimistic as long as she avoids stress and alcohol. As long as she continues to take Free and Easy Powder in extract I believe she will not experience any further dysplasia or the growth of any neoplasm either in her pelvis or her breasts. Had she not sought and received effective treatment for her constellation of symptoms, Chinese medical theory would definitely prognose the likelihood of her developing cancer at some point in the future.

Case #3: A woman 34 years old complained of PMS, the major symptom of which was a migraine headache at ovulation and on the first day of her period. The headaches was a one-sided temporal headache accompanied by nausea and chills. The day before the headache her neck and shoulders became very tense. Her other PMS symptoms included moodiness, lower abdominal bloating, breast tenderness, and a craving for sweets and chocolate. Her menstrual cycle was regular and she had a bright, healthy discharge with no cramping. The patient had cold hands and feet and sometimes could hear water sloshing in her Stomach. She had a tendency toward vaginitis. She had previously had a history of cystitis. Eleven years ago she had two cysts removed, one from her breast and the other from under her arm. She had two children, aged 12 and 9. Seven years ago she had her tubes tied. Her tongue was skinny, a little purplish, and had a normal coat, although the surface of the tongue appeared moist. Her pulse was thready and wiry and bilaterally weak and deep at the Foot position.

Her Chinese diagnosis was Liver Qi Congestion, Blood Deficiency, and Water Stagnation in her Stomach. I prescribed Free and Easy Decoction with increased doses of Atractylodes and Poria and the addition of Alisma to remove the Stagnant

Water. Two days before the onset of her period and the anticipated date of her next migraine she received acupuncture at Gallbladder 20 (*Feng Chi*), Gallbladder 14 (*Yang Bai*), Gallbladder 8 (*Shuai Gu*), Gallbladder 41 (*Zu Lin Qi*), and Triple Heater 5 (*Wai Guan*), all on the left side only, and Conception Vessel 12 and Stomach 40 (*Feng Long*), bilaterally. The unilateral points were selected to prevent her headache by opening up the *Shao Yang Luo Mai*. The bilateral points were selected to remove the Stagnant Water in her Stomach. Two days later the patient did have a headache which was 25% lighter and shorter than usual and not accompanied by nausea or chills. Acupuncture at the same unilateral points with the substitution of Triple Heater 3 (*Shou Lin Qi*) for Triple Heater 5 with the electrical stimulation of Triple Heater 3 and Gallbladder 41 followed by *Tuina* massage completely eliminated any residual pain at the tail end of the headache.

Following this headache the patient's formula was revised to place more emphasis on dredging the Liver and destagnating the Blood in the *Luo Mai*. Cortex Radicis Moutan, Fructus Gardeniae, Herba Menthae, Flos Carthami, Radix Ligustici Wallichi, and Radix Platycodi were added to her formula. Her next headache was two days earlier than expected. Therefore, the patient did not receive any preventive acupuncture. Instead she came for treatment during the headache. She was needled at the same points as her last treatment plus the addition of an *Ah Si* point on her left temple. 80% of her discomfort was relieved within fifteen minutes. The needles were removed and the remaining 20% of the pain was relieved by *Tuina*.

After this the patient switched to Xiao Yao San, the patent medicine pills with Moutan, Gardenia, and Mint. Her next headache was very light and she did not seek treatment for it. Her premenstrual symptoms in general were much improved. She was advised to continue taking the pills for several more months to consolidate the therapeutic results.

One interesting aspect of this case was that this woman's headaches began after moving to Colorado from sea level. Most migraines in women are due in part to Blood Deficiency. It is my theory that her Blood Deficiency only became apparent when she moved to a higher altitude where there is an increased demand placed on the red blood cells. It is also possible that the *Feng Shui* or Geomancy of this area, which includes a preponderance of Wind energy, aggravated her Liver. I have had several other female patients who only developed migraines after moving to Colorado.

CASE #4: A woman 38 years old complained of anxiety, depression, frustration and anger during her premenstrual period. She did not complain of breast swelling, bloating, menstrual irregularity, or cramps. She did complain of frequent colds and migraine headaches which were sometimes associated with her period and sometimes not. She had some tinnitus but no dizziness. She had nocturia and dry skin but no palpitations. She said she was very fatigued lately and that she had used a lot of "recreational" drugs in the past. The patient had never had any children. She was a musician and therefore travelled a lot and kept irregular hours and diet. Her tongue was deeply fissured and had been for at least twelve years. It was also somewhat red. Her pulse was a little slow or relaxed on the right hand but its size and depth were ok. On the left hand the pulse was thready and wiry, especially so at the Gate position. Both Foot positions were deep and weak.

Her diagnosis was Liver Qi Congestion with Blood and Kidney Deficiency. I prescribed Xiao Yao Wan patent medicine and Kidney Nourishing Pills, also a proprietary medicine. After two months the patient reported that her nocturia was improved, her periods were totally cramp-free, and that her energy was much better. She did not feel so cold and the warmth in her hands and feet was consistently improved. Her mood seemed perhaps better, but she still overreacted to stress.

At this point the patient had an upper respiratory tract infection which she had for three weeks while "on the road". She had sore throat, thick green phlegm, and a cough. The patient had a headache and felt subjectively hot. Her temperature, taken orally, was 36 degrees Centigrade. Her tongue had a thick yellow coat and her pulse was thready overall but fast on both right and left Inch positions. I prescribed Zhi Shou Ding Chuan Wan patent pills for Hot Phlegm in the Lungs and applied acupuncture to Lung 5 (*Chi Ze*) and 7 (*Lie Que*), Bladder 13 (*Fei Shu*), Large Intestine 20 (*Ying Xiang*), and Gallbladder 20.

The patient registered marked improvement but four days later complained of a dry unproductive cough in the evenings and sore throat mornings and evenings. The patient exhibited malar flushing and reported that her face felt red. Her tongue looked "baked" red. Her pulse was fast, thready, and wiry. Her diagnosis was Lung & Kidney Yin Deficiency. I administered acupuncture at Lung 7, Kidney 6, Bladder 13, Lung 1 (*Zhong Fu*), Lung 10 (*Yu Ji*), and Small Intestine 17 (*Tian Rong*) and prescribed Ophiopogon Decoction, 2 *bao* per day according to the doses in *Commonly Used Chinese Herb Formulas With Illustrations* with the inclusion of 10 grams wild American Ginseng. The patient took this formula for several days and received a second acupuncture treatment consisting of Lung 7, Kidney 6, Small Intestine 17, and Bladder 52 (*Zhi Shi*).

For the next month this patient had relapses of chronic sore throat alternating with periods of moodiness and anxiety. During this period she took Free and Easy Decoction with the addition of Ophiopogon, Raw Rehmannia, and Scrophularia to moisten her Yin. Her next period was cramp-free with a

30

healthy, fresh menstrual flow. By this time the patient was not experiencing any migraines. Her skin was moister and her urination less frequent.

The patient felt that her moodiness, depression, and anxiety were no longer associated with her menstrual cycle. From the point of view of PMS, she felt that any symptoms related to her period were improved. However, she still complained of frustration and anger which were out of proportion to their external stimuli. In analyzing her symptoms further I discovered that the patient's "sore throat" was actually a sensation of constriction. I also learned that she held within her a great deal of suppressed anger at her parents. While the patient was lying on the examination table, I jiggled her abdomen and elicited the sound of sloshing water in her Stomach. Based on this I prescribed Pinellia and Magnolia Combination, classically known as the Decoction of Four and Seven, which is indicated for Congested Liver Qi at the level of the throat and Stagnant Water in the Stomach.

I no longer consider this patient a PMS case even though her diagnosis is Constrained Liver Qi due to anger. Rather than administering acupuncture on an on-going basis, I recommended that she receive short-term psychotherapy to help her deal with the suppressed anger directed at her parents. This anger was not simply historical but the patient was continuing to generate fresh anger based on past experiences. She was unable to let go and forgive and forget. This case is an example that one must not become rigid in the prescription of a Chinese formula based on a Western diagnosis but must constantly re-analyze difficult cases and alter prescriptions as necessary. It also points to my belief that personality problems based on the false notion of the separate ego cannot and should not be treated by such external remedies such as herbs and acupuncture but require personal growth. Chinese medicine can treat the secondary cause of disease, i.e. humoral and energetic imbalance, but it cannot treat the primary cause which is our existential dilemma. This ultimately is a spiritual dilemma which can only adequately be addressed on that level.

Case #5 A 29 year old woman presented multiple complaints which she did not identify as PMS. She experienced depression, anxiety, frustration, and suicidal moods. Her period was regular but her flow had gotten progressively shorter and she passed a lot of large clots the first couple of days each month. Her periods were also becoming more and more painful each month. He breasts were very sore. She had colds hands and feet, some dizziness, and some palpitations. She was not married and had no pregnancies or abortions. Five years ago she had colitis. She still had irregular bowel movements, fluctuating from constipation to diarrhea. Often she experienced pain in her lower right abdomen. She also felt a tight constriction in her chest and her breath was shallow. Besides her other complaints, the patient had chronic vaginitis, herpes genitalia, and vaginal warts. Her tongue was a light purplish brown. The fur was white, thin, and moist to the front and yellow tinged with brown to the rear. Her pulse was fast. Her left pulse was markedly finer than her right and both Foot positions were tight at the Human level.

Her diagnosis was Liver Qi Congestion with Spleen Deficiency. I prescribed Bupleurum and Cinnamon Combination in powdered extract. She took this for ten days and developed hematuria. I then prescribed Minor Bupleurem Combination and Hoelen Five Herb Formula. Within two days here urine returned to normal. She complained of feeling premenstrual and of loose bowels with mucous clumps. She switched back therefore, to the Bupleurum and Cinnamon Combination. Also she complained of a heavy vaginal discharge. In addition to the herbs, I inserted needles at Liver 3, Spleen 6, Stomach 36, Conception Vessel 6, and did moxa at Conception Vessel

12 and Stomach 25. Within two days the mucous in her feces was gone but her bowels were still loose. I did acupuncture at Liver 3, Spleen 6, Conception Vessel 6, and Pericardium 6 and moxaed Stomach 36 and Conception Vessel 8 (*Shen Que*). Three days later the patient reported healthy, well-formed stools with no mucous. She was still depressed but felt much better for a day or so after each acupuncture treatment. On this day I needled Liver 3, Spleen 6, Pericardium 6, Conception Vessel 6, and Stomach 29.

After that period I switched the patient to Free and Easy Powder in extract, 2 grams 3 times per day. She took the herbs regularly and registered considerable improvement over five months. Her breasts no longer became swollen. Her cramps were less. Her blood flow was fuller, i.e. back to normal, although she still passed some clots. The month after she had received acupuncture she had not passed any. She felt much more stable but she still had a lot of leukorrhea. Her bowel movements were consistently healthy and regular.

Over the next month I treated this patient primarily for leukorrhea with both herbs and acupuncture. The leukorrhea was thick and varied from white to yellow. When it became yellow it also smelled bad. Her tongue was a little swollen and moist and had a red tip. Its coat was thin and white with a little cracking in the center. Her pulse was thready and wiry. The patient also experienced a fairly consistent one-sided headache following the course of the Gallbladder meridian. Her acupuncture consisted of needling Triple Heater 3, Gallbladder 41, Gallbladder 26 (*Dai Mai*), Conception Vessel 6, Spleen 6, Stomach 36, Bladder 23 (*Shen Shu*) and Bladder 32 (*Ci Liao*). As an herbal formula I prescribed Free and Easy Powder with the addition of Rehmannia. This variation is called Black Free and Easy Powder. By the end of the month her leukorrhea was considerably improved and her headache was gone.

Three months later this patient had a car accident which produced a lot of stress and she went off her diet. She also drank more alcohol to which she was very sensitive. Her bowels became loose and a little mucousy and she was afraid her colitis was returning. One acupuncture treatment returned her stools to normal. The points used were Stomach 36, Spleen 6, Liver 3, Stomach 25, Conception Vessel 12, and Pericardium 6.

Five months after that she still had some loose stools, breast tenderness, one-sided headache, and vaginal discharge. Her tongue was a little flabby. Its color was good and the cracking in the center was much less. Her right pulse was wiry and a little thready. Her left pulse was thready and a little wiry. I prescribed a Decoction for Ending Leukorrhea which she took for approximately one month. After this her discharge was much better and her period was "real gentle". However, her bowels had become loose again. Her tongue was palish and a little swollen. I prescribed the Decoction of Six Gentlemen plus Free and Easy Powder both in extract form.

The patient had no further problems with premenstrual or menstrual-related symptoms for over six months. Then, due to a stressful living and family situation, she let her anger get out of control. Her stools became loose; her breasts got tender; her one-sided headache returned; and her vagina began to itch. She also had sores in her mouth, bleeding gums, and bad breath. Her tongue was purplish and puffy with a red tip. Her pulse was full and wiry. She received several acupuncture treatments from another acupuncturist while I was in retreat. Points used included Liver 2 (*Xing Jian*), Gallbladder 41, Stomach 25, Spleen 6, Stomach 44 (*Nei Ting*), and Large Intestine 4. When I returned a couple of weeks later, she reported that she felt 100% better but that she was urinating more frequently, experiencing some terminal dribbling, and was dizzy when she stood up. Her left Foot pulse was definitely

34

weak. I needled Bladder 52 for ten minutes with tonification.

This patient exemplifies the sometimes cyclic or recalcitrant nature of Liver Qi Congestion when it is complicated by Heat and Dampness harbored in the Lower Burner. Although she always responded to treatment and over the two years she has been receiving Chinese herbs and acupuncture has made overall improvement, her tendency is to fall back into old patterns under stress and for her bowels to become disordered every Fall. This points out the diligence and perseverance necessary to effect lasting and fundamental change in deep-seated personality related problems such as Liver Qi Congestion.

It is important to understand that a patient does not *have* Liver Qi Congestion but *is* Liver Qi Congestion. This disharmony is a problem in the way in which a person is, is with her or himself, and is with reality at large. It is questionable in my mind whether, without a program of sophisticated and time-tested disciplines and skillfully administered psychoemotional stimuli, a person can really change who they fundamentally are in one lifetime. Many New Age growth therapies seem to be to substitute one style of being for another but do not radically change the structure of the ego itself. As mentioned in case #4, it is my belief that Chinese medicine cannot radically effect such change either. There is a limit to what herbs and acupuncture can do and this necessitates seeing and dealing with the problem of life and the ego from a higher, i.e. spiritual perspective. However, for dealing with the physical and clinically significant emotional discomfort caused by Liver Qi Congestion, Chinese herbs and acupuncture are effective.

One of Chinese medicine's great assets is its ability, through the application of its theories, to progress a disease into the future and show its probable effect on the other organs and mechanisms of the body. Liver Qi Congestion, as mentioned above, first typically weakens the Spleen through the *Ke* or

35

Control cycle according to Five Element theory. This leads to faulty digestion and an impaired production of Qi and Blood. Spleen and/or Qi and Blood Deficiency are not terminal patterns in Chinese medicine, but Liver Qi Congestion and Qi and Blood Deficiency lead to an easy production of Stagnant Blood. Also stated above, there are three regions of the body where Stagnation of Liver Qi tends to manifest in the female. These are the pelvis, breasts, and throat. Stagnancy in the first two of these typically causes neoplasms which may become malignant. If such neoplasms are treated by surgery without correcting the underlying Stagnation, this Stagnation will simply manifest in some other area of the body. If the breast is removed it may often lead to tumors in the pelvis. If a hysterectomy is performed, this may lead to Splenomegaly. If the Spleen is removed, this may often be followed by cirrhosis of the Liver or Liver cancer and life cannot be preserved without a Liver. In other cases, if the Spleen is removed pancreatic cancer may develop which is likewise terminal.

Therefore, the treatment of PMS is important in order to prevent more serious diseases later in life. If we are seeing an epidemic of PMS now, in ten to fifteen years we will see an epidemic of breast and pelvic neoplasms in these same women according to Traditional Chinese Medicine. This epidemic can be averted if the Liver Qi Congestion is relieved before it becomes substantial Blood Stagnation. The treatment of Liver Qi Congestion by Chinese medicine is relatively simple and successful even though the causes of this pattern of disharmony are deeply rooted in our contemporary society. I believe Chinese medicine, in fact, has the clearest and most efficacious description of the cause and cure of this malady and that it can help alleviate the suffering of literally millions of American women.

APPENDIX

Ingredients of the herbal formulae mentioned in the text:

Decoction of Four and Seven

Rhizoma Pinelliae
Cortex Magnoliae
Fructus Perillae
Sclerotium Poriae Cocoris
Fructus Ziziphi Jujubae
Rhizoma Recens Zingiberis

Minor Bupleurum Combination

Radix Bupleuri
Radix Codonopsis Pilosulae
Radix Scutellariae
Rhizoma Pinelliae
Fructus Ziziphi Jujubae
Rhizoma Recens Zingiberis
Radix Glycyrrhizae

Four Ingredient Decoction

Radix Angelicae Sinensis
Radix Rehmanniae Conquitae
Radix Paeoniae Albae
Radix Ligustici Wallichi

Bupleurum and Cinnamon Combination

Radix Bupleuri
Rhizoma Pinelliae
Ramulus Cinnamomi

Radix Paeoniae Albae
Radix Glycyrrhizae
Radix Scutellariae

Radix Codonopsis Pilosulae   Rhizoma Recens Zingiberis
Fructus Ziziphi Jujubae

Dang Gui Sixteen Herb Combination

Radix Angelicae Sinensis   Radix Astragali Seu Hedusari
Ramulus Cinnamomi   Cortex Magnoliae
Radix Platycodi   Fructus Perillae
Radix Linderae   Radix Paeoniae Albae
Radix Saussureae Seu Vladimireae   Semen Arecae
Radix Glycyrrhizae   Radix Angelicae
Radix Ligustici Wallichi   Fructus Aurantii Immaturi
Radix Codonopsis Pilosulae   Radix Ledebouriellae

Ophiopogon Decoction

Tuber Ophiopogonis   Radix Codonopsis Pilosulae
Rhizoma Pinelliae   Radix Glycyrrhizae
Fructus Germinatus Oryzae Sattivae
Fructus Ziziphi Jujubae

Decoction for Ending Leukorrhea

Rhizoma Atractylodis Macrocephalae Rhizoma Atractylodis
Radix Dioscoreae   Radix Glycyrrhizae
Radix Codonopsis Pilosulae   Pericarpium Citri Reticulatae
Radix Paeoniae Albae   Herba Seu Flos Schizonepetae
Semen Plantaginis   Radix Bupleuri

Decoction of Six Gentlemen

Radix Codonopsis Pilosulae   Fructus Ziziphi Jujubae
Rhizoma Pinelliae   Radix Glycyrrhizae
Rhizoma Atractylodis Macrocephalae
Pericarpium Citri Reticulatae
Sclerotium Poriae Cocoris   Rhizoma Recens Zingiberis

38

ENDNOTES

1   Kaptchuk, Ted, *The Web That Has No Weaver* (Congdon & Weed), NY 1983, p. 179-180

2   *Common Terms Of Traditional Chinese Medicine In English* (Beijing Medical College), Beijing, 1980, p. 14

3   Ibid. p. 14

4   Ibid. p. 75

5   "The Liver & Gallbladder", ed. & trans. by C.S. Cheung & Jenny Belluimini *Journal of The American College of Traditional Chinese Medicine*, San Francisco, #2, 1983, p. 35

6   Li Ke Shao, "Insomnia: Historical Review of Differential Diagnosis and Treatment", *Journal of ACTCM*, #3, 1984, p. 35

7   *Common Terms* etc., op. cit. p. 20

8   Lu Gwei Djen & Needham, Joseph, *Celestial Lancets, A History And Rationale of Moxa* (Cambridge University Press), Cambridge, etc. 1980, p. 27-39

9   Zhuan Zi, *Zhuan Zi Ji Shi*, edited by Guo Qing-fan, (Zhong Hua Shu Ju), Beijing, 1982

10   Hsu Hong-yen & Hsu Chau-shin, *Commonly Used Chinese Herb Formulas With Illustrations* (Oriental Healing Arts Institute), Los Angeles, 1980, p. 87

11   "Traditional & New Interpretations of Prescriptions", trans. & ed. by C.S. Cheung & Jenny Belluomini,

JACTCM, #1, 1984, p. 8-11

12   Hsu & Hsu, op. cit., p. 537

CERVICAL DYSPLASIA

Due to the introduction of the Papanicolaou test, the so-called Pap smear, many women today are diagnosed as having cervical dysplasia. Cervical dysplasia is the presence of abnormally growing cells on the cervix. This is considered a precancerous condition and depending upon the severity of the dysplasia, cauterization, cryosurgery, or excision are typically recommended by allopaths to kill or remove these aberrant cells. Biopsies are likewise often performed either separately or in conjunction with the above-mentioned procedures. Pap smears allow for this early detection of such a precancerous condition. As such they have saved countless lives. Many women who are in otherwise seemingly good health from the point of view of allopathy are apprised of something amiss in their pelvis before a tumor or palpable neoplasm actually arises. However, from the point of view of Traditional Chinese Medicine, the allopathic therapies currently used to treat cervical dysplasia themselves aggravate and complicate the underlying cause of the dysplasia. At the very least, they fail to reverse the underlying process which produces the dysplasia. Traditional Chinese Medicine, on the other hand, has available to it extremely effective therapies which have no iatrogenic complications. In addition, Chinese medicine not only eliminates the symptom of dysplasia but corrects the underlying energetic imbalance responsible for the dysplasia. Since the taking of a Pap smear is a relatively benign procedure, this is one instance where an allopathic diagnostic technique when wedded to a Traditional Chinese Medical treatment results in a very fortuitous cure.

Western allopathic medicine clinically contents itself with the destruction of any abnormal cells found on the cervix. Scant attention is paid preventively to why the body has created or allowed the growth of such cells. Cauterization or excision of such cells may remove them temporarily but it does not, in my experience, abort the process of their production. Without correcting or negating this process it is likely that such cells will be produced again. Or, if the cauterization or excision has made it impossible for this process to manifest as cervical dysplasia, it may perforce manifest in a predictable, at least according to Traditional Chinese Medical theory, as some other, usually neoplastic pathology.

Traditional Chinese Medicine describes most neoplasms as "Stagnations" of one sort or another. According to Chinese medicine, various energies and substances circulate through the body over discrete and identifiable routes. If one or more of these energies becomes blocked it will tend to pool behind the blockage causing a localized stagnation. Zhu Dan-xi of the Jin-Yuan ennumerated the Six Stagnations. They are pathologic accumulations of Qi (vital energy), Blood, Dampness, Fire, Phlegm, and Food.[1]

Of these six, the first two are usually considered the most important and, in fact, have a mutual relationship. It is said that the Qi moves the Blood as part of its *Yun Hua*, transportation and transformation, function. If the Qi becomes stagnant, over a period of time the Blood normally "pushed" by the Qi will also become stagnant. On the other hand, since the Blood is the material basis of the Qi[2], if the Blood is obstructed

42

the Qi will also stagnate.

In the clinical practice of traditional Chinese gynecology, Stagnant Qi and Stagnant Blood are commonly encountered energetic etiologies responsible for many female complaints. Definite diagnostic criteria exist for the differential diagnosis of these two patterns of disharmony. For instance, based on signs and symptoms, tongue, and pulse, the experienced practitioner is able to distinguish between dysmenorrhea due to Stagnant Qi and dysmenorrhea due to Stagnant Blood. Although for clarity's sake, especially in teaching, these two patterns of disharmony are presented as discrete energetic entities, in truth there exists a continuum from free-flowing Qi and Blood through Stagnant Qi to Stagnant Blood. Stagnant Blood can also be differentiated relatively into insubstantial and substantial degrees. Insubstantial Stagnant Blood is defined as the conceptual organization of a group of signs and symptoms referred to theoretically as Stagnant Blood. Substantial Stagnant Blood refers to the palpable or visible presence of a pathological mass or to ecchymosis or extravasation. It is interesting to note that in Chinese medicine all pain is due to Stagnation. Stagnation may be due to an excess of Qi or Blood, to the presence of an obstructing and inappropriate energy such as Dampness or Cold, or to a Deficiency of Blood retarding the flow of Qi.

By the time a woman is diagnosed by Western medicine as having a tumor or neoplasm in her pelvis Chinese medicine would often diagnose her as suffering from Stagnant Blood. However, in the case of cervical dysplasia where a tumor or mass has yet to form, the typical Chinese diagnosis is not Stagnant Blood but Stagnant Qi or, in some cases, borderline Stagnant Qi/Stagnant Blood. This is a relatively happy state of affairs since Chinese medicine regards Stagnant Qi as easier to treat than Stagnant Blood. Such Stagnant Qi can be treated either by herbs or acupuncture, but, in my experience, when

43

herbs and acupuncture are combined together with proper dietary and lifestyle modifications, the overwhelming majority of cervical dysplastic cases can be reversed within three months as evidenced by subsequent negative Pap smears.

However, before such efficacious treatment can be implemented we must further describe and define where and why this Qi has become Stagnant. In Chinese, the *Xue Shi*, the Blood Chamber, refers to both the Liver and the Uterus.[3] In fact, in Traditional Chinese Medicine, the word *Gan*, usually translated as Liver, does not mean liver in itsWestern biological sense but rather an energetic configuration which includes both the liver and the uterus within it. In other words, the Chinese terms *Gan* and *Xue Shi* could be considered synonyms which stand for a single energetic entity, parts of which are variously referred to as the liver and uterus. In my experience, women who have cervical dysplasia as diagnosed by positive Pap smears suffer from Liver Qi Congestion. This may or may not mean that their Western liver function as diagnosed by blood analysis is out of the ordinary. This means, from the Chinese medical point of view, there is a congestion or stagnation of energy in the *Gan* which includes the liver, the uterus, the hypochondrium, the intercostals, and parts of the throat, gingiva, eyes, and head. Congestion of Liver Qi may manifest in any or all of these areas of the body traversed by the *Jue Yin* and *Shao Yang* meridians which arise from or are intimately connected with the Chinese concept of the *Gan*.

Liver Qi Congestion may be due to a number of factors. I have described these at length in "Premenstrual Syndrome (PMS): Its Differential Diagnosis and Treatment" appearing in the *American Journal of Acupuncture*, Vol. 13 No. 3, July - September 1985. Briefly, however, the Liver energy becomes congested primarily due to psychoemotional stress. As is said in Chinese, *Gan Wei Gang Zang:* the Liver is the Organ of temperament.[4] Unrestraint of the Seven Passions has a strong

44

unbalancing effect on the Liver since the Liver's function is to spread the Qi and therefore the emotions in a smooth and moderate way. In Chinese, the word Qi not only means energy but it is also used to describe a person's emotional state. Therefore we can say a person's Qi is angry if they look upset. In particular, the Liver is easily and negatively affected by anger in all its various permutation, including frustration. The negative effects of anger, frustration, and stress in general on the Liver are aggravated by improper diet, trauma of any kind to the areas traversed by the *Gan* or its channels, and any interference with the body's biological clock regulated by the diurnal and seasonal progression as they manifest at a specific place on the planet.

Foods which tend to aggravate Liver Qi Congestion are coffee; alcohol; greasy, fried, and fatty foods; spicy, pungent, and acrid foods; heavy, hard-to-digest foods; chemical preservatives; and drugs; and over-eating in general. Of these, coffee is perhaps the most specific and detrimental food for a person suffering from Liver Qi Congestion and should be avoided entirely. Trauma to areas traversed by the meridians and channels associated with the Liver include tubal ligations, abortions, biopsies, cryosurgery, and C-section. Latent Damp Heat and Toxins in the Foot *Jue Yin* meridian, suppressed but not eliminated by antibiotics, as in the allopathic treatment of venereal disease, can also cause or add to Liver Qi Congestion, especially as it manifests at the level of the Lower Burner. Interference with the biological clock harming the smooth, regular, and appropriate flow of Qi includes high speed, long distance travel hopscotching time zones and even seasons and the use of hormones as in birth control pills. All these things in my experience, adversely affect the patency of Liver Qi. In female patients, Liver Qi most often manifests in the Lower Burner or pelvis as one or another gynecological complaint. Cervical dysplasia is one of these.

When the Liver Qi becomes congested this often causes imbalance in the Spleen as well. Just as the Traditional Chinese Medical Liver is not the Western biological liver, the Spleen or *Pi* is not the biological Spleen. The Chinese concept of Spleen includes the spleen and pancreas and to some extent includes the entire process of digestion. According to Five Phase theory, when the Liver becomes Excess, which it does when it is congested, this Excess may be vented on the Spleen through the *Ke* or Control cycle. This typically causes a weakening of the Spleen. When the Spleen becomes weak, digestion will be impaired; there may be diarrhea or constipation; and the production of Blood will be inhibited. Therefore, in clinical practice, most women who suffer from Liver Qi Congestion likewise show some signs of Spleen Deficiency complication as well.

When the Spleen becomes weak, it may also and often does lose its ability to transport and transform Water in the body. This results in a certain amount of Dampness accumulating internally. This Dampness may first accumulate in the Spleen itself, thus affecting digestion, but it will eventually spill over into the body at large. Since Dampness is "heavy", it tends to seep down from the Middle to the Lower Burner where it accumulates. As mentioned above, Dampness may itself become a source of Stagnation. Dampness impedes the flow of Qi. Because Qi is inherently Warm energetically, Heat is absorbed from the blocked Qi by the Dampness thus transforming into pathological Damp Heat. Damp Heat in the Lower Burner is therefore often the result of Liver Qi Congestion and Spleen Deficiency *cum* Dampness and in turn causes further obstruction of the Qi and Blood in the pelvis. In the same way, Stagnant Blood absorbs Heat from the Qi and may transform into Stagnant Heat and Blood. Over a period of time this pathological Heat will tend to exhaust the Yin and the Blood.

Since the hemopoietic activity of the Spleen is typically impaired by Congested Liver Qi, various symptoms of Blood Deficiency as described by Traditional Chinese Medicine, may be seen in patients with this scenario. As the Blood becomes "thin" or "dry" it all the more readily absorbs Heat from the Congested Qi. This is especially so since the Blood is believed to be stored in the Liver according to Oriental theory. This then can lead to various symptoms due to Hot Blood. It is the Blood which moistens and nurtures the Liver. As the Blood becomes Dry, the Liver becomes Hotter. This tends to exhaust the Kidney Yin since the Liver and Kidney share a "common source". Since the Essence of the Liver and Kidney can reinforce each other, Deficiency of the one will result in Deficiency of the other.[6] Then, since Kidney Yin and Yang are mutually reciprocal and because the Spleen will seek reinforcement from the Kidney Yang, the Kidney Qi is likely to be weak in such patients as well. All these relationships, complications, and permutations must be kept in mind when diagnosing and erecting a Traditional Chinese Medical treatment plan for a patient whose Western allopathic diagnosis is cervical dysplasia.

In general, I have achieved very good results in treating cervical dysplasia by adopting a similar treatment plan to that used in treating PMS and dysmenorrhea. In fact, most women who receive a diagnosis of cervical dysplasia subjectively suffer form one of these two complaints and only more rarely from both. In cases where the patient does suffer from pronounced premenstrual symptoms and severe dysmenorrhea, the degree of Stagnation is more severe and the Five Phase and Humoral complications are more complex. The basis of my treatment of cervical dysplasia is a Chinese herbal formula which dates from the Sung dynasty: Xiao Yao San. This is the first formula I usually think of when treating a woman with Liver Qi Congestion, Spleen Deficiency, and gynecological symptoms. Depending upon the presenting signs and symptoms and the congestion, Spleen Deficiency, and gynecological symptoms. Depending upon the presenting signs and symptoms and the patient's condition and constitution, I then modify this formula by appropriate additions and deletions. This formula and its applications and modifications have been discussed in some detail elsewhere.[7, 8, 9, 10] Usually the patient is required to take this prescription in decoction for from two to three menstrual cycles.

As an adjunct to such herbal therapy I usually administer acupuncture every other day before the onset of menstruation beginning six to eight days before the expected due date. Although the selection of the points depends again upon the fine points of the diagnosis and the presenting symptoms, I often begin my choice from a standard group of points: *Tai Chong* (Liv 3), *San Yin Jiao* (Sp 6), *Xue Hai* (Sp 10), *Guan Yuan* (CV 4), *Gui Lai* (St 29). *Tai Chong*, the *Yuan* Source point of the Liver meridian dredges Stagnant Qi by tapping into the *Yuan Qi*, the aspect of the Qi responsible for its motility. *San Yin Jiao* improves the circulation of the Qi and Blood in the pelvis in general. *Xue Hai* deobstructs Stagnant Blood and cools the Blood[11] and therefore indirectly cools and relaxes the Liver. *Gui Lai* moves Stagnation of Qi and Blood and removes Blood stasis from the uterus.[12] And *Guan Yuan* regulates the Qi[13], especially the *Yuan Qi* and especially vis a vis menstruation.[14] All these points are needled with reduction technique after having obtained the Qi and the needles are left passively in place for typically twenty minutes.

Women who, due to distance or schedule, cannot receive such premenstrual acupuncture are usually advised to do a ginger compress on their lower abdomen every evening for twenty minutes beginning approximately one week before their period. Acupuncture and such compresses are employed during this phase of the cycle since it is at this point that the Qi and Blood are pooling in the pelvis. This is when congestion is most likely and manipulation. And this is when the body itself is preparing to rid itself of any toxicity and Stagnation through the menstruation. Acupuncture during the first half of the cycle is not cost-or-time-efficient since the Qi is moving up and away from the pelvis[15] and since the main priority of the body at that time is the production of Blood, not its dispersal.[16]

Adequate exercise to circulate the Qi and Blood and rest to reduce and relax tension are highly recommended lifestyle modifications for patients with cervical dysplasia due to Liver Qi Congestion. Since "lack of physical exercise or necessary physical exertion may cause retardation of Qi and Blood,"[17] a sedentary lifestyle logically tends to augment Stagnation of Qi originally caused by stress and/or trauma. Programmed deep relaxation can reduce stress and its negative effects at their source. However, to accomplish this it must be practiced consistently over a period of time until one has been habituated to the technique and can apply it successfully throughout the day.

The following case histories illustrate typical medical histories and presenting signs and symptoms of American women I have treated with cervical dysplasia.

Case #1: The first case is of a woman thirty-two years old. The patient had used an IUD for three years ten years before her first visit to me. She had tried several different kinds, including the infamous Dalkon Shield, each one causing her either physical discomfort, menorrhagia, or dysmenorrhea. She had suffered from herpes genitalia for seven years, usually experiencing one outbreak per month. She had had two abortions one and two years before she was first diagnosed as having cervical dysplasia. Four months before coming to me she had undergone cryosurgery for dysplasia. The dysplasia had reappeared and her gynecologist again suggested the same procedure. She suffered from PMS beginning at ovulation with lumbar pain, a bloated lower abdomen, swollen and tender breasts, and irritability and depression. Her periods were regular and without much cramping but her discharge tended to be dark, dryish, and somewhat clotty. Her cycle was short at twenty-three days. The patient had one bowel movement per day. Her stools tended to fall apart and sometimes contained undigested food. She was fatigued and chilled easily but did not have habitually chilled hands and feet. Her tongue was a bit flabby but not fluted, with a thin white coat. The color was a bit pale and slightly brownish. Her pulse was fastish, fine, and wiry, especially on the left. My diagnosis was Stagnation of Qi in the Lower Burner due to Liver Qi Congestion, Occluded Damp Heat in Lower Burner, and Spleen Dampness.

The patient received three or four acupuncture treatments in the week before her period for three cycles. Since she typically complained most of depression and breast tenderness, her acupuncture treatments usually consisted of *Tai Chong, San Yin Jiao, Gui Lai, Qi Hai* (CV 6), *He Gu* (LI 4), *Nei Guan* (Per 6), and sometimes *Shan Zhong* (CV 17). At the time of treating this woman several years ago I did not have access to custom modified bulk herb prescriptions. Therefore I suggested Jia Wei Xiao Yao Tang in powdered extract. I suggested she avoid Liver-aggravating and Spleen-weakening foods. Foods which cool the digestion and aggravate Dampness are raw fruits and vegetables, cold or chilled foods and drinks, and excessive liquids in general. In particular, this patient had craving for coffee, chocolate, and ice cream which she was cautioned to abstain from as completely as possible. I also suggested she practice deep relaxation for twenty minutes per day every day for a minimum of six weeks. The patient was reasonably athletic and received adequate exercise already.

The first period after beginning treatment the patient passed a more than usual amount of dark, clotty blood. She also experienced more than usual cramps on the first day of her period. Although her diagnosis was not Stagnant Blood per se, still there was some Stagnant Blood associated with the Stagnant Qi in her pelvis. The discharge of dark clots with more intense cramping the first and/or second periods after beginning treatment should be taken as a good sign that the Stagnation of Qi and Blood is being dispersed and discharged. Her second and third periods showed consistently more and fresher blood and her cycle lengthened to twenty-eight days.

Because the patient continued to indulge her coffee and sweet addiction and because of various emotional upsets in her life, like breaking up with her boyfriend, she continued to require one or two acupuncture treatments per period to relieve her sore breasts and depression. After six months of taking Jia Wei Xiao Yao Tang, her bowel movements were consistently more formed and she was no longer fatigued. At that point she got a new Pap smear which was negative. Three years later, although the patient still experiences infrequent outbreaks of herpes and occasional premenstrual emotional lability if she indulges in coffee, chocolate, or ice cream, further Pap smears have all been negative.

Case #2: This woman was 26. Since menarche this patient had always had severe cramps on the first day of each period. Sometimes the pain was accompanied by vomiting and hyperventilation. Up until the preceding nine months the patient's cycle had been regular at twenty-eight days. For the last nine months it had been consistently one week overdue. For two and a half months prior to her first visit the patient had had a thick creamy, white, and itchy vaginal discharge. The patient came to me because she had recently received an irregular Pap smear. Two Western allopaths had suggested she have cryosurgery within the next six months. In addition, the patient experienced stabbing pain with intercourse seventy per cent of the time, had varicosities on the backs of her knees, experienced hemorrhoids once in a while, and vaginitis at least once per year. When she was twenty she had been treated with Flagyl for an ovarian cyst. Her mother had had a hysterectomy and a history of severe dysmenorrhea. The patient's bowel movements were normal. Her tongue had a pronounced red tip with a thin white coating. Her pulse was wiry at the left *Guan* and deep and wiry at the left *Chi*. My diagnosis was Stagnant Qi and Blood in the Lower Burner due to Liver Qi Congestion and Congenital Stagnant Blood.

My choice of prescription for this patient was Xiao Yao Tang with the addition of Corydalis, Cyperus, Saussurea, Salvia, and Carthamus. The formula was administered in decoction, the added ingredients chosen to increase the formula's effect on destagnating specifically the Blood. Acupuncture was administered at *Tai Chong, He Gu, San Yin Jiao, Xue Hai, Guan Yuan,* and *Gui Lai* three times in the week before each of the next three periods. At the end of that time, the patient's cycle was back to twenty-eight days; she experienced only light diffuse cramps; did not experience pain with intercourse; and her discharge was bright and fresh and of a moderate amount. At this point she again had a Pap smear which was negative.

Seven months later the patient's menstruation was still regular and unproblematic. Then, due to job-related stress, she experienced loose stools with undigested food, lower abdominal cramping and bloating, fitful sleep, and Plum Seed Qi or neurotic esophageal stenosis. Her tongue was fluted and pale with the same pronounced red tip extending two fifths of the way back from the apex. Abdominal palpation revealed Water Stagnation in the Stomach. Her pulse was superficial on the right and larger on the left. Both *Chi* were deep. My diagnosis was Wood Invading Earth with Liver Qi Congestion the throat and Stagnant Water in the Stomach. I prescribed four doses of Ban Xia Hou Pu Tang in decoction which alleviated all the patient's symptoms. This second development shows how Liver Qi can manifest in another area of the body and how persistent this imbalance is.

Case #3: The third case is of a thirty-five year old woman. She had had very irregularly lengthened cycles for the last four months. She had received two irregular Pap smears and had been diagnosed as having benign atypical dysplasia. Her MD had suggested a biopsy. Her menstrual discharge was thinner and more mucousy than before with less clotting. Previously, her first day's discharge was heavy, dark, and clotty. The degree of cramping was usually related to the amount of exercise she received. Since she had not been exercising lately due to business stress, her cramps were lasting longer and her periods were fatiguing. She had lots of neck and shoulder tension. Premenstrually her breasts had been tender the last three to four months and she had been depressed throughout this period of time. She was typically constipated, and a chronic headache over the right eye, and was sometimes nauseous when anxious. Her vaginal discharge had changed in the last few months becoming more abundant, stronger smelling, and yellowish but not curdy.

The patient was the mother of a thirteen year old, had had one abortion at nineteen, and at twenty-one had given birth to a non-surviving preemie due to placenta abruptio. She had also had a fibroid removed form her breast at around nineteen. Her tongue was paleish and purplish, fluted and fat, with a red tip and a thin white coat. Her pulse was thready, deep, and relaxed on the right. On the left it was similar except for being wiry on the *Guan* and *Chi*. My Chinese diagnosis was Liver Qi Congestion with Spleen Damp and Deficient Heat.

For this patient I created two separate versions of Jia Wei Xiao Yao Tang[19]. The first was modified with the addition of

Codonopsis, Cooked Rehmannia, Orange Peel, and Green Orange Peel. This was administered in decoction for the first fifteen days of the cycle to tonify the Deficiency and seep the Dampness from the Middle. During the second fifteen days of the cycle, Corydalis, Cyperus, and Saussurea were added to the formula to destagnate the Qi and Blood. This patient declined acupuncture due to her busy schedule. After two months of this regime all her symptoms were relieved and her Pap smear was normal. She continued to take Xiao Yao Wan in patent pill form for another couple of months to consolidate the therapeutic results. I suggested that because of this woman's busy and stressful professional life she continue these pills for even another six months. However the patient was too busy to remember to do this and I expect to see her again for the same or a related problem in the future. In general, I like to see my patients continue their therapy, if only in patent pill form, for as much as one month for every year they have suffered from a tendency to Liver Qi Congestion. In this case since she was nineteen years old.

Case #4: The fourth case is of a twenty year old. Four months prior she had had an irregular Pap smear. She went back the next month and received the same result. The following month she had had a biopsy. Her MD recommended cryosurgery. The patient had been on birth control pills for six years. Before that she had had severe dysmenorrhea. Her mother and grandmother had likewise suffered from dysmenorrhea. While on the Pill she did not experience cramps and her discharge was heavy only the first day and clot free. She did experience some premenstrual emotional lability. Her hands and feet were typically cold. The consistency of her stools fluctuated. Drinking coffee usually resulted in loose stools. Her tongue was slightly fluted and definitely had a red tip. The coat was yellow and greasy to the rear. Her pulse was relaxed in pace, a bit wiry on the right *Guan*, and deep on the right *Chi*. Her left *Guan* was threadier and her left *Chi* deeper, threadier, and more wiry still. This patient experienced pain on palpation in the substernal area and pain at *Huang Shu* (Kid 16). She also had a pronounced descending aortic pulse abdominal conformation. My diagnosis was Liver Qi Congestion and Imbalance of the *Chong* and *Ren* channels.

Since the patient did not intend to stop taking birth control pills at that time, I felt I could only prescribe for the presenting symptoms. Therefore I administered unmodified Xiao Yao Tang in decoction. Since the patient had minimal presenting signs or symptoms besides the positive Pap smear, I did not suggest acupuncture. After one month the patient decided to give up the Pill at which time I deleted Ginger and Mint from her formula and added Corydalis, Cyperus, Saussurea, Persica, and Salvia. She began this modified formula after midcycle. Her period was only slightly painful and she discharged a lot of purplish black clots. The next month I prescribed Xiao Yao Tang minus Mint and plus Codonopsis and Cooked Rehmannia to tonify for the first half of the cycle and then Xiao Yao Tang without Ginger and plus Cyperus and Corydalis to disperse Stagnation during the second half. This period was painless with a healthy, clot-free discharge. The patient then received a negative Pap smear and consolidated her therapeutic result be taking Xiao Yao Wan in patent pill form for four more months.

In the last few years I have averaged about six cases of cervical dysplasia per year. Almost all have achieved negative Pap smears after three or four months of the treatment outlined above. Only one patient has received a positive Pap smear since the time of concluding her therapy and one month's additional treatment was all that was required to reverse that again. Therefore, I consider cervical dysplasia to be highly amenable to Traditional Chinese Medical treatment. However, several points should be noted. Xiao Yao San and the

55

acupuncture points given above are not specific treatments for the allopathic diagnosis of cervical dysplasia. The practitioner of Traditional Chinese Medicine must still diagnose each case of dysplasia in Chinese medical and energetic terms and the treatment plan must be logically derived from that diagnosis. I have written this paper only to suggest that, in my experience, the traditional Chinese diagnosis for patients with cervical dysplasia has been consistently some version of Liver Qi Congestion.

Although I have treated successfully mild, moderate, and severe dysplasia, I have not had as simple a time with patients suffering from carcinoma in situ. Although this is only a further progression in this scenario, five and six months of consistent herbal and acupuncture therapy, although achieving considerable amelioration in signs and symptoms, have not as yet achieved a negative Pap smear. Therefore, although I believe that the treatment of carcinoma in situ is possible with Traditional Chinese Medicine, it is my advice that the practitioner make a more guarded prognosis and expect a more protracted period of therapy than in cases of dysplasia.

Gynecology or *Fu Ke* is one of the specialties of Traditional Chinese Medicine which really shines in comparison with Western allopathy. Not only are traditional Chinese gynecological treatments effective but traditional Chinese diagnosis makes much more sense of our patients' medical histories and the constellation of their signs and symptoms. Traditional Chinese Medical theory explains energetically why the vast majority of gynecological problems arise, and not only that, but, based on that theory, the practitioner can also prognose the likely development of an energetic imbalance if that imbalance's symptoms are merely suppressed. Cervical dysplasia, *if it devolves into a malignancy,* usually results in a hysterectomy. Since a hysterectomy does not and cannot stop the progressive development of Liver Qi Congestion in other

56

areas of the body, if more women with dysplasia were treated with Traditional Chinese Medicine, far fewer hysterectomies would be performed. This in turn would result in fewer mastectomies, splenectomies, and thyroidectomies down the line and fewer deaths from cancer in general among women. Without Pap smears, many women would not realize that, in fact, something is clinically amiss in their pelvis until a neoplasm or substantial Stagnant Blood arises. Therefore, practitioners of *Fu Ke*, traditional Chinese gynecology, should welcome the advent of the Papanicolaou test.

ENDNOTES

1   *Common Terms Of Traditional Chinese Medicine In English*, by committee, (Beijing Medical College), Beijing, 1980, p 55

2   Ibid. p. 45

3   Ibid. p. 14

4   Ibid. p. 20

5   Ibid. p. 20

6   Ibid. p. 21

7   Cheung, C.S. & Belluomini, J., "Traditional and New Interpretations of Prescriptions: The Harmonizing an Relieving Group", *JACTCM*, SF, #1, 1984, p. 8-11

8   Hsu, Hong-yen & Hsu, Chau-shin, *Commonly Used Herb Formulas With Illustrations*, (OHAI), LA, 1980, p. 94-5

9   Yeung, Him-che, *Handbook of Chinese Herbs and Formulas*, Vol. II, LA, 1985, p. 263

10 Flaws, Bob, "Premenstrual Syndrome (PMS): Its Differential Diagnosis & Treatment", *AJA*, Vol 13, #3, Jul.-Sept. 1985, p. 211-12

11 Maciocia, Giovanni, "The Actions of the Points", a collection of reprints from the *Journal of Chinese Medicine*, issues 1-6, England, p. 9

12   Ibid. p. 8

13   *Acupuncture: A Comprehensive Text,* by committee, Shanghai College of Traditional Chinese Medicine, Trans. & Ed. by John O'Connor & Dan Bensky, (Eastland Press), Chicago, 1981, p. 185

14   Ibid. p. 12

15   Darras, Jeanne Claude, "The Genital System", xeroxed reprint distributed by OICS, CA as part of their on-going education for graduates, p. 5-10

16   After menstruation the woman tends to be relatively Blood Deficient.

17   *Essentials Of Acupuncture,* by committee, Beijing College of TCM, Shanghai College of TCM, Nanjing College of TCM, & The Acupuncture Institute of the Academy of TCM, (Foreign Language Press), Beijing, 1980, p. 46

18   Ingredients in Ban Xia Hou Pu Tang:
        Rhizoma Pinelliae
        Cortex Magnoliae
        Folium Perillae
        Sclerotium Poriae Cocoris
        Rhizoma Recens Zingiberis

19   Ingredients in Jia Wei Xiao Yao San:
        Radix Bupleuri
        Radix Angelicae Sinensis
        Radix Paeoniae Albae
        Radix Atractylodis Macrocephalae
        Sclerotium Poriae Cocoris

PELVIC INFLAMMATORY DISEASE (PID)

Pelvic Inflammatory Disease or PID is a commonly encountered problem in contemporary clinical practice. However, in my opinion, it is not a problem which allopathic medicine treats very satisfactorily. This is due to Western medical theory's blind spot concerning this disease. By definition, PID is seen by allopaths as a bacterial infection in the pelvis. The basic allopathic treatment for bacterial infection is antibiotics. However, in my experience and according to Traditional Chinese Medical theory, what we call PID is not necessarily or only due to infection by microbial pathogens. Since Western allopathic theory is limited by its emphasis on microbial infection, it fails to erect a comprehensive treatment plan for patients suffering from PID which takes into account other factors besides the killing of bacteria. Chinese medicine, on the other hand, describes what we call PID as any of three basic patterns of disharmony which take into account not only the presence of pathogens but also the internal environment of the individual. Because of Chinese medicine's more comprehensive theory concerning the pathophysiology of this disorder, it sees PID patients with both greater resolution and more holistically. It is my experience that Chinese medicine treats PID very effectively, especially in terms of long-term complications. Although Chinese medical treatment for PID usually stretches over a longer period of time than with Western allopathy, it is capable of arresting the tendency to chronic relapse characteristic of antibiotic therapy.

According to Traditional Chinese Medicine, the three patterns of disharmony which most frequently correspond to the Western diagnosis of PID are Toxic Heat Accumulating in the Lower *Jiao*, Stagnant Qi and Blood in the Lower *Jiao*, and Deficient Spleen and Kidney Qi.[1] Although for teaching purposes these three patterns are presented as three distinct conceptual entities, in my experience, most PID patients present a combination of these patterns. In fact, these three patterns represent a continuum. Toxic Heat Accumulating in the Lower *Jiao* represents the acute, inflammatory phase of this disease. Stagnant Qi and Congealed Blood describes both the underlying chronic pattern of disharmony which creates the environment in which Toxic Heat can accumulate and also the chronic, recalcitrant post-acute pattern following antibiotic treatment. Deficient Spleen and Kidney Qi is a pattern often complicating Stagnant Qi and Congealed Blood. It also represents both the serious iatrogenic complications of excessive antibiotic therapy and the end result of a patient suffering from chronic PID over a long period of time.

Toxic Heat Accumulating in the Lower *Jiao* is characterized by acute onset, systemic fever, lower abdominal pain which resists pressure, yellow, thick, and purulent vaginal discharge, low back pain, frequent or rough urination, lack of appetite, nausea, dry mouth, constipation, a red tongue with yellow fur, and a wiry, rapid pulse. Most of these signs and symptoms corroborate the flourishing of Toxic Heat which corresponds to infection. Antibiotics are extremely Cold in nature and antitoxic. Therefore they can neutralize the Heat and Toxicity of inflammation according to TCM heteropathic logic. However, the wiry pulse, nausea, lack of appetite, and the name of the pattern which includes the concept of Accumulation all suggest that more than Heat and Toxicity should be addressed in this situation.

Toxic Heat, when it accumulates in the Lower *Jiao*, causes an impediment to the free flow of Qi and Blood in that area. This in turn causes or aggravates Stagnant Qi and/or Blood. Since this area is irrigated by the Liver, this may cause or aggravate Liver Qi Congestion. It is this Liver Qi Congestion venting on the Spleen which causes the nausea and lack of appetite. Antibiotics do nothing to redress the Stagnation caused by the accumulation of Toxic Heat nor to harmonize this Liver and Spleen. When antibiotics are given orally, they typically cause diarrhea due to their chilling of the Spleen Yang. Even when given intravenously, they tend to depress the body's Yang and therefore depress the *Zheng Qi*, the Righteous Qi associated with immunity. Therefore, defining this problem as only an inflammation due to infection without regard to the vigor of the *Zheng Qi* and the patency of the Qi and Blood leads to a treatment which is completely ineffective for the two other patterns of disharmony diagnosed by Western allopaths as PID and only partially effective for this first pattern.

In my experience, antibiotic treatment alone for this first type of PID *leads* to the two subsequent patterns of disharmony. The acute Heat and Toxicity are neutralized but a chronic Stagnant Qi and Congealed Blood pattern is created. Most often there is a pre-existing chronic Liver Qi problem. This pre-existing condition creates the environment for the Heat and Toxicity to flourish in the first place. This remains and is aggravated by the antibiotic treatment. Typically, patients treated solely by antibiotics have recurring bouts of PID. The antibiotics, by depressing the Righteous Yang at the same time as neutralizing the Evil pathogens tend to weaken the Spleen. This directly affects the production of Postnatal Qi and Blood. Weakening the Spleen Qi causes poor digestion. This is turn leads to weakness of the Blood and the generation of Internal

Dampness. As the Spleen becomes weak, the Liver may become both more congested and hotter. Liver congestion leads to poor circulation in the pelvis and especially in the Uterus. Heat in the Liver meridian in this area combines with Dampness dripping down from the Spleen. This Heat and Dampness, when they accumulate, transform into Toxic Heat and the patient may experience an acute flare-up of their infection. If, however, there is not much Heat or Dampness being generated by the Liver and Spleen respectively, the patient will tend to experience symptoms of the second patterns of disharmony.

Stagnant Qi and Congealed Blood in the Lower *Jiao* is a chronic problem. The Stagnant Qi refers to Stagnant Liver Qi. The Congealed Blood may be either substantial or insubstantial. The symptoms of this pattern are: lower abdominal and hypogastric pain, stabbing pain or a falling feeling in the lower abdomen, low back pain, possible discharge, either white or slightly yellow but thickish, a possible palpable mass in the hypogastrium, either a pale or darkish tongue, possible red papillae, white or yellow fur depending upon the amount of Dampness or Heat, and a wiry, sunken, thready, and/or astringent pulse. The permutations of this pattern are numerous depending upon the relative strengths and weaknesses of the Five *Zang*, the Qi and Blood, the Yin and Yang, and the presence of various pathologic substances such as Dampness and Stagnant or Congealed Blood. This pattern and its permutations are what I most commonly encounter in my practice and antibiotics, as stated above, do little if anything but make this pattern more chronic and recalcitrant.

In women with this pattern of disharmony, the diagnostic label Pelvis Inflammatory Disease is a misnomer. Most of the symptoms are not due to inflammation or infection but to Stagnation. Since Western allopathy does not have such a theoretical concept, it cannot see such patients clearly. Western MDs, when they cannot find any sign of infection in such women by pelvic examination resort to the expensive and invasive procedure of laparoscopy. This is the insertion of a fiber optic through an incision in the navel to seek out an infection in the endometrium. Often this likewise turns up no sign of an infection. In my experience, many MDs will still insist that the patient has PID even when no sign can be found. Since this is the only theory Western medicine has to account for these symptoms, it must insist on its rectitude even when it cannot find justification for this theory in an individual patient. When I asked an allopath why he thought Western medicine handles this problem so ineffectively, he said that it is because there are so many different possible pathogenic bacteria that it is often difficult to prescribe the correct specific antibiotic. This is the so-called silver bullet theory of medicine. This belief that there is a specific pathogen which can be killed by a specific antibiotic only leads Western clinicians away from seeing the patient as a whole.

Liver Qi Congestion with Stagnant Blood in the Blood Chamber seems to be reaching epidemic proportions in the American female population between twenty and thirty years of age. This is due to a large number of factors including psycho-sociological stress, abortions, C-sections, antibiotic treatment of urogenital infections, tubal ligation, tampons, intercourse during menstruation, hormone-based birth control, etc. I have discussed some of these factors at greater length in "Premenstrual Syndrome (PMS): Its Differential Diagnosis & Treatment"[2] and "Cervical Dysplasia: Its Diagnosis & Treatment According to Traditional Chinese Medicine"[3]. The more one understands the Liver's role in traditional Chinese pathophysiology, the more easily will one be able to identify all the complications and permutations of Liver-related disorders. These go beyond the scope of this present work. However, American practitioners of Chinese medicine are mentioning

65

more and more frequently the preponderance of Liver-related disharmonies in their patient populations.[4]

The third Chinese pattern of disharmony sometimes diagnosed in women who have also been diagnosed as having PID is Deficient Spleen and Kidney Qi. In this pattern the Pre and Postnatal Qi have been seriously weakened. All the symptoms are due to Deficiency of the *Zheng Qi*. They are: clear, watery leukorrhea, lumbar soreness, lower abdominal soreness which feels worse after exertion or intercourse, fatigue, edema in the lower legs, orthostatic hypotension, cold hands and feet and a desire for warmth, frequent urination, and diarrhea or watery stools. The tongue is pale with a white coating. The pulse is frail and soggy. Since from the Chinese medical point of view the treatment principle for this type of PID is to tonify the Righteous, any attacking of supposed Evils, for instance by antibiotics, will cause a further worsening of the patient's overall condition.

This pattern is not as frequently met with, in my experience, as the preceding one. When I have seen this pattern, it has been in women who have either suffered from chronic PID for a very long time or who have been extremely exhausted by antibiotic therapy. When such patients are tonified, they often will develop more acute symptoms or stronger abdominal pain. This may happen for either of two reasons. If, after tonification, they exhibit symptoms corresponding to Toxic Heat, it is because their *Zheng Qi* had previously been too weak to battle the Excess Evil. Inflammation is a battle. If the Righteous Qi is too weak to mobilize such a battle, the infection will become latent only to be reactivated when the environment has enough energy to support it. If, on the other hand, the tonified patient does not experience Toxic Heat symptoms but rather pain more characteristic of Stagnant Qi and Blood, it is because previously there was not enough Qi and Blood flowing through the obstructed passageways to experience the potential blockage. Once the Qi and Blood are raised from a trickle to normal volume, constraint or blockage of the channels and collaterals will be experienced as pressure, i.e. pain.

When either of the above scenarios present, this is not a sign of further deterioration. Rather they are indications of the return of the *Zheng Qi*. In the case of Toxic Heat, there is now Righteous Qi which can be mobilized to attack and eliminate the Evil Toxins. In the case of Stagnation of Qi and Blood, there is now enough Qi and Blood to direct towards the Stagnation to crack it and sweep it away. This should be carefully and patiently explained to the patient in some detail in order to gain her trust and insure her perseverance in the treatment. In cases without signs of Heat or Toxicity, one does not need, in my experience, to be overly concerned about spreading infection within the pelvis creating adhesions, abscesses, or scar tissue. If the Chinese-style therapy eliminates the pain *and* all other parameters return to normal, such as menstrual discharge, regularity, digestion, energy level, vaginal discharge, etc., one can assume that the patient's internal environment has also returned to normal. If there are signs of Heat and Dampness or Toxicity according to the diagnostic signs and symptoms of Chinese Medicine, care must be taken and judgement exercised so that complications do not occur. This may mean even resorting to antibiotics to contain and quickly neutralize a virulent and spreading infection. If such antibiotic treatment is combined with Chinese-style treatment to disperse Stagnation, dry and seep Dampness, and tonify the *Zheng Qi*, especially of the Spleen and Kidneys, the infection will not get out of hand *nor* will a significant aspect of the problem be left untreated.

Chinese medical treatment is effective even in cases of strong Heat Toxin PID. Herbal formulae such as Long Dan Xie Gan Tang[5] (Decoction to Purge Liver Fire with Gentiana) can be administered orally. Such Reducing formulae should only be administered, however, for a few days. If and as the patient exhibits signs that her *Zheng Qi* is becoming weak, such as Spleen Deficiency diarrhea, they must be modified in order to protect and nurture the patient's Righteous Energy. She Chuang Zi Chong Xi Ji[6] (Decoction of Cnidium Fruit for Vaginitis) can be used as a vaginal douche. These two herbal treatments should be supplemented by acupuncture treatment given once or even twice per day. Point selected will depend on the individual's presenting symptoms and the relative proportions of Righteous and Evil Qi. The points I am most prone to employ are *San Yin Jiao* (Sp 6), *Xue Hai* (Sp 10), *Fu Liu* (Ki 7), *Qu Quan* (Liv 8), *Gui Lai* (St 29), and *Guan Yuan* (CV 4). *San Yin Jiao* mobilizes and regulates the circulation of the pelvis. *Xue Hai* destagnates the Blood and cools Heat associated with the Blood. *Fu Liu* tonifies the Kidneys but also clears and cools Damp Heat.[7] *Qu Quan* clears and cools Damp Heat in the pelvis, especially from the Foot *Jue Yin*. *Gui Lai* is a local point for destagnating Qi and Blood in the lower abdomen. *Guan Yuan* is a crossing point of the Foot Three Yin which locally destagnates Qi and Blood and regulates the *Zheng Qi* of the pelvis through the medium of the *Yuan Qi*. The needles should be manipulated with strong Reducing technique to the limits of the patient's tolerance and left *in situ* for a relatively long period of time up to one hour.

In the majority of PID cases corresponding to Stagnant Liver Qi and Congealed Blood, I typically use Xiao Yao Tang[8] (Free and Easy Decoction) as the basis of an orally administered herbal prescription. Usually I modify this standard formula with Moutan and Gardenia and also Salvia, Capillaris, Taraxicum, Persica, and/or Leonurus depending upon the situation. If Heat and Dampness are significant, i.e. if there is a yellow discharge, I usually include Capillaris and Taraxicum. If Stagnant Blood is more significant, I am likely to add Persica, Salvia, and/or Leonurus. Since, as stated above, the permutations of this stage or type of generally chronic or recalcitrant PID are so large in number, the number of potential modifications are likewise large and other formulae altogether may also be more appropriate. Xiao Yao Tang is, however, a good basic formula since is tonifies Qi and Blood, disperses Dampness, activates Qi and Blood, and harmonizes the Liver and Spleen. In the chronic or recuperative stage of this disorder, some amount of all these principles is usually indicated.

Since vaginal discharge is usually not purulent with this basic pattern, I do not usually prescribe a douche. Acupuncture is useful but less frequently and less forcefully. When PID is chronic I usually administer acupuncture every other day during a flare-up. Since such flare-ups typically occur during premenstrual build-up, I routinely schedule three or four treatments during that time during the first month or cycle of treatment. This is to diminish pain and to take advantage of the body's natural movement towards discharge at this time. Qi and Blood are at their maximum in the pelvis at this time. Therefore, just as at the Full Moon systemically, this is the time to disperse locally. Points selected again vary depending upon the individual pattern. However, typical points employed include *Tai Chong* (Liv 3), *San Yin Jiao, Xue Hai, He Gu* (LI 4), *Gui Lai*, and *Guan Yuan*. *Tai Chong* and *He Gu* in combination are called the Four Gates. They open the flow of Qi and Blood in the entire body. *He Gu* in particular sends the Qi down into the pelvis in order to mobilize the Blood for discharge.

In my experience, two or three months of consistent treatments for this type of PID with custom-blended herbal prescriptions and acupuncture usually achieve a satisfactory result. Success is determined based on the diminishment of pain in the lower abdomen, normalization of the menstrual cycle, normalization of the menstrual discharge, and elimination of any vaginal discharge. During these three months, it is important that the patient modify her diet, emotions, and lifestyle similar to the recommendations I have given for the treatment of PMS.[9] If we accept the idea that disease is a teaching from reality that something is wrong in the way we are pursuing our lives, then the treatment of PID should take into account these other factors. Most of my PID patients, it seems to me, have gone through periods of unrestrained lifestyle. If the patient is willing to take responsibility for her imbalance and accept the behavioral implications of Chinese energetic theory, she will get the full value out of her investment in herbs and acupuncture. If, on the other hand, the patient sees no relation between her lifestyle and her disease but rather views her problem as an adventitious imposition, she will probably not see her treatment through to successful completion. Successful Chinese-style treatment for PID, it seems to me, requires a certain maturity on the part of the patient and implies that the healer must be as much a teacher and counselor as an administrator of technical intervention.

In women suffering from chronic and recalcitrant PID due to Spleen and Kidney Deficiency, there are likely to be emotional complications. When the Spleen and Kidneys become weak there is a lack of Will and sense of fear which makes it difficult for such patients to be patient. Since the Spleen and Kidneys are intimately connected with the production of Blood, the Blood in such patients tends to be Deficient. The Blood Deficiency fails to nourish and support the *Shen* in the Heart and these patients may have difficulty holding on to a consistent treatment plan and realistic chronological treatment goals. There are several formulae that I typically chose from with such patients, such as modified versions of Gui Pi Tang[10], Shih Quan Da Bu Tang[11], Ba Zhen Tang[12], etc. If both Pre and Postnatal energies are depleted, it is often difficult for the body to assimilate the herbs and catalyze a return to health. Often times a small dose is more easily assimilable and effective than a larger dose. I have also noticed that such patients often are too nervous to accept acupuncture treatment. In such patients, moxibustion is preferable and indicated and other non-threatening, home remedies such as ginger compresses. All too often, such patients, captivated by their fear, return for more antibiotics which only make their condition worse in the long run. A great deal of support, nurturance, explanation, and patience are required when dealing with such patients.

Case History: A woman twenty-nine years old and single

Two weeks before coming to me she had been diagnosed by an allopathic physician as having PID. She had been given Penicillin and Flagyl simultaneously. Her symptoms had cleared up for two days but then returned. Her physician wanted her to go back on antibiotics, perhaps intravenously as an in-patient in the hospital. One month previously she had experienced mid-cycle bleeding which had lasted for one week. At that time her doctor had diagnosed cystitis since there was blood in her urine and she had had a long history of recurrent bladder infections. The patient also had a history of yeast infections and herpes genitalia. For the past year she had had increasing dysmenorrhea. Her cycle was irregular, tending to be short, sometimes in fact having a period every two weeks. Her menstrual discharge was dark with black clots. Four years ago the patient had had abdominal pain and her doctor had suggested exploratory surgery which she declined. She had had one miscarriage and her sister had similar dysmenorrhea. In addition, the patient experienced premenstrual soreness of the breasts, edema, fatigue, emotional lability, and depression. Since the PID, her period pain was "unbearable". At the time of her first visit she did not have a fever or a vaginal discharge. She did experience constant pain over both ovaries. She was very fatigued and had diarrhea from the antibiotics. Her tongue had a red tip, was small and pale, and a little moist. Its coating was yellow to the rear. Her pulse was soft, deep, and weak on the right and thready on the left with the left *Chih* being thready, deep and wiry.

My diagnosis was Stagnant Qi and Blood, Liver Qi Congestion, and Deficient Spleen Qi. I made tonification of the *Zheng Qi* my primary goal with some destagnation of the Blood. The prescription I wrote was:

Radix Angelicae Sinensis	9 grams
Radix Paeoniae Albae	9 "
Rhizoma Atractylodis Macrocephalae	9 "
Sclerotium Poriae Cocoris	9 "
Radix Codonopsis Pilosulae	9 "
Radix Astragali Seu Hedysari	12 "
Radix Praeparatus Glycyrrhizae	6 "
Cortex Radicis Moutan	6 "
Radix Salviae Miltorrhizae	6 "
Radix Rehmanniae	9 "

This was to be taken in decoction over a two day period. I also administered acupuncture at *Tian Shu* (St 25), *Gui Lai, Zu San Li* (St 36), *San Yin Jiao, Xue Hai, Fu Liu, Pi Shu* (Bl 20), and *Da Chang Shu* (Bl 25).

By the next day the bowel movements and stools had returned to normal. After the previous day's treatment the pelvic pain had subsided. However, the next day it returned seemingly more intense. Therefore I concentrated the acupuncture on the Stagnation in the pelvis. Her treatment that day consisted of *Gui Lai, Guan Yuan, San Yin Jiao, Xue Hai,* and *Tai Chong.* The patient was expecting her period in the next day or so. Again the pain backed off only to return more intense and sharper the next day. I interpreted this as the Qi and Blood trying to crack the Stagnation. Therefore, the next day I again administered the same acupuncture treatment as the day before but wrote a different herbal prescription:

Semen Persicae	9 grams
Flos Carthami	9 "
Apex Radicis Angelicae Sinensis	9 "
Radix Ligustici Wallichi	6 "
Radix Paeoniae Rubrae	9 "
Radix Paeoniae Albae	9 "
Radix Praeparatus Glycyrrhizae	6 "
Radix Rehmanniae	6 "
Rhizoma Cyperi	9 "
Rhizoma Corydalis	6 "
Myrrha	6 "
Radix Saussureae Seu Vladimiriae	6 "

Again this was to be taken in decoction over a two day period.

The following day the patient's period had still not come. She experienced pelvic pain on and off and I administered the same acupuncture treatment. The next day her period did start but she did not have the intense sharp cramps she had had the last couple of periods. Her discharge was a fresh, bright red. I decided not to administer any further acupuncture at that time but changed her formula to the following:

Radix Bupleuri	9 grams
Radix Angelicae Sinensis	9 "
Radix Paeoniae Albae	9 "
Radix Ligustici Wallichi	9 "

73

Radix Praeparatus
          Glycyrrhizae   6 "
Rhizoma Atractylodis
          Macrocephalae   9 "
Sclerotium Poriae Cocoris   9 "
Rhizoma Cyperi   9 "
Rhizoma Corydalis   6 "
Myrrha   6 "
Radix Saussureae Seu
          Vladimiriae   6 "

The dosage was the same as above.

Two days later the patient reported some intense cramping the day before but no sharp, stabbing pain. The cramping was localized over her left ovary. Her blood flow was clear with no clots. On the present day she did not experience any cramping at all. Since women are typically Blood Deficient immediately after their periods and since this patient's *Zheng Qi* had not yet recuperated from her illness and the antibiotics, I decided to prescribe modified Shih Quan Da Bu Tang to tonify her Qi and Blood up until ovulation. The formula was:

Radix Astragali Seu
          Hedysari   9 grams
Cortex Cinnamomi   6 "
Radix Codonopsis Pilosulae   9 "
Radix Rehmanniae
          Conquitae   12 "
Rhizoma Atractylodis
          Macrocephalae   9 "
Sclerotium Poriae Cocoris   9 "
Radix Angelicae Sinensis   9 "
Radix Paeoniae Albae   9 "
Radix Ligustici Wallichi   6 "
Radix Praeparatus

Glycyrrhizae	6	"
Radix Saussureae Seu		
Vladimiriae	6	"
Fructus Seu Semen Amomi	6	"

One *bao* was to last two days and I gave her two *bao*[13]. Five days later the patient reported feeling much stronger. She still, however, felt some dull pain in the lower left abdomen. I added 6 grams of Salvia and 9 grams of Leonurus to the above formula and gave her five more *bao*. Ten days later the patient reported passing ovulation and that the pain in her lower abdomen was returning. Therefore, I prescribed the following Blood-destagnating formula to be taken through her period:

Radix Bupleuri	6 grams	
Apex Radicis Angelicae		
Sinensis	9	"
Radix Paeoniae Albae	9	"
Radix Paeoniae Rubrae	9	"
Radix Ligustici Wallichi	6	"
Rhizoma Atractylodis		
Macrocephalae	9	"
Sclerotium Poriae Cocoris	9	"
Radix Praeparatus		
Glycyrrhizae	6	"
Herba Leonuri	9	"
Feces Trogopterori Seu		
Pteromi	6	"
Rhizoma Corydalis	6	"
Radix Saussureae Seu		
Vladimiriae	6	"

After the next period, the patient reported no PMS symptoms and no period pain. She said that her period was the best she had had in years. However, she still experienced some continuous mild pain in her lower abdomen. Once again I modified her formula to emphasize the chronic nature of the soreness. The patient also had to be encouraged to continue and was told, in fact the end was in sight. Her formula at this point consisted of:

Radix Angelicae Sinensis	9 grams
Radix Ligustici Wallichi	6 "
Radix Paeoniae Rubrae	9 "
Fructus Foeniculi	3 "
Rhizoma Corydalis	6 "
Feces Trogopterori Seu Pteromi	6 "
Myrrha	6 "
Cortex Cinnamomi	6 "
Rhizoma Dessicata Zingiberis	6 "
Pollen Typhae	6 "
Radix Codonopsis Pilosulae	9 "
Radix Rehmanniae Conquitae	12 "
Gelatinum Asini	6 "

The next time the patient reported in was ten days before her next period. She felt great. The pain had completely disappeared and her energy felt back to normal. There were no PMS symptoms and the patient was very pleased. She asked if she could discontinue the herbs since she felt so well. I advised her to continue on the same formula through her next period, which she did. This period likewise was very good. After her period, I suggested she continue taking Xiao Yao Wan patent pills for several months to consolidate her result. Since the causes of PMS, PID, and Liver Qi Congestion are so numerous and endemic in our society, given this woman's history, it is likely that she may experience some Liver-induced problems in the future. This is especially so since she did not really come to understand or appreciate Chinese medicine's philosophy on her situation. This was, perhaps, due to my reticence and failure as a teacher. However, six months later the patient has not experienced any recurrence of abdominal pain, dysmenorrhea, or premenstrual tension.

Many female patients ask, and rightfully so, how long they will have to take Xiao Yao Wan. This is a difficult question to answer. All too often, after several months of taking Xiao Yao Wan and then several months of not, some Liver Qi induced problem arises. This may be a relapse of the initial problem or may be a different set of Liver-related symptoms such as the woman I treated last summer for endometriosis and this winter for hiatal hernia. Commonly, women with Liver Qi Congestion also manifest a wiry pulse. I have never felt such a pulse ever lose its wiry quality even after several years of off and on therapy for Liver-related disorders. This is distressing to patients and to myself as well. It is important that all parties in the healing endeavor recognize that Liver Qi Congestion is not something one has but rather *is*. As stated in other articles, it is my belief that the endemic prevalence of Liver Qi Congestion disorders in American women between the ages of twenty-five and forty is due to the unnatural stress of our society and environment.

It seems to me that we as humans are not coping with all the myriad stressors in our contemporary lives. In fact, I am coming to the conclusion that without a radical change in the patient's lifestyle it is impossible to effectively deal with Liver Qi Congestion at its root. If a radical reorientation of lifestyle and personality are not undertaken, the best Chinese medicine can do is to cope with the various clinical problems caused by Liver Qi Congestion, such as PMS, PID, cervical dysplasia, breast cancer, etc. Although Chinese medicine, acupuncture and herbs, do effectively treat the diseases caused by Liver Qi Congestion, they are not enough to neutralize the pervasive and debilitating stressors in our modern life which cause this condition.

This is a problem that Chinese medicine in America must come to terms with. Modern American society is vastly different from even contemporary Chinese culture, not to mention classical Chinese culture. In a traditional culture, episodes of stress causing Liver Qi Congestion may not be that uncommon, but still they are episodic. Here, our level of comparatively intense stress is continuous and unrelieved. Anyone who has not lived in a Third World country may have difficulty understanding just how stressful our lives are. Chinese medicine in America must address this difference in its approach to therapy, especially preventive therapy. In my opinion, American practitioners will have to make more conscious and copious use of lifestyle counselling and adjunctive therapies such as deep relaxation, biofeedback, massage, etc. than commonly encountered in Chinese clinics. Although Chinese herbal medicine is not meant to be taken as a perpetual supplement like Western vitamins, still American women suffering from various Liver Qi disorders may have to remain on formulae such as Xiao Yao Wan for prolonged periods of time unless they are able and willing to make major lifestyle adjustments. Because of our culture's pervasive stress and the frustration inherent in stress, modern practitioners of Chinese medicine may have to once again conceive of themselves primarily as teachers and counsellors and secondarily as acupuncturists and herbalists.

ENDNOTES

1   Kaptchuk, Ted, *The Web That Has No Weaver*, NY 1983, p. 332-333

2   Flaws, Bob, "Premenstrual Syndrome (PMS): Its Differential Diagnosis & Treatment", *American Journal Of Acupuncture,* Felton, CA, Sept, 1985, Vol. 13 #3

3   Flaws, Bob, "Cervical Dysplasia: Its Diagnosis & Treatment According to Traditional Chinese Medicine", *Journal Of The American College of Trad. Chin. Med.,* SF, #4, 1985

4   Lee, Peter Bing Heng, "Liver Ailments According to the Five Element Theory", *Pacific Journal of Oriental Medicine,* Summer 1985, Vol 2 #2

5   Ingredients of Long Dan Xie Gan Tang: Gentiana, Scutellaria, Gardenia, Alisma, Plantaginis, Akebia, Raw Rehmannia, Dang Gui tails, Bupleurum, and Licorice

6   Ingredients of She Chuang Zi Chong Xi Ji: Fructus Cnidii Monnieri, Sophora, Melia, Phellodendron, Cortex Lycii Radicis, and Alum

7   Anon. Committee, Shanghai College of Trad. Chin. Med., *Acupuncture: A Comprehensive Text,* ed. & trans. by John O'Connor & Dan Bensky, Chicago 1981

8   Ingredients of Xiao Yao Tang: Bupleurum, Atractylodes, Poria, Dang Gui, Peony, Ginger, Treated Licorice, and Peppermint

9   Flaws, "Premenstrual Syndrome", op. cit.

10   Ingredients of Gui Pi Tang: Ginseng, Astragalus, Dang Gui, Atractylodes, Saussurea, Poria, Polygala, Zizyphus Spinosa, Zizyphus Sattiva, Treated Licorice, and Ginger

11   Ingredients of Shih Quan Da Bu Tang: Astragalus, Cortex Cinnamomi, Ginseng, Cooked Rehmannia, Atractylodes, Dang Gui, Peony, Cnidium, Poria, and Treated Licorice

12   Ingredients of Ba Zhen Tang: Ginseng, Cooked Rehmannia, Atractylodes, Dang Gui, Peony, Cnidium, Poria, Treated Licorice, Ginger, and Zizyphus Sattiva

13   *Bao* is the Chinese word for packet. One *bao* therefore is one packet of herbs. Prescriptions are administered per *bao*.

HAN BAI LING ON THE PREVENTION OF MENSTRUAL DISORDERS AND THE IMPORTANCE OF LIFESTYLE MODIFICATION IN THE AMERICAN PRACTICE OF ORIENTAL MEDICINE

When a patient comes to an American acupuncturist with a disease or disorder with which the practitioner has had no previous experience, he or she is likely to look up the disorder in such basic formularies as *Comprehensive*[1] or *Essentials*[2]. Basing a treatment plan on the information provided, the American practitioner often will not achieve the results implied by such Chinese discussions. Acupuncture treatment plans as given in the two above mentioned texts are predicated upon treatments administered three times per week. Most American practitioners and their patients find this schedule economically unfeasible. However, this is not the only nor the main reason why American patients do no respond to Chinese-style therapy the way Chinese do.

Zhang Yuan-su in the twelfth century suggested that remedies which worked in one time and place may not be effective in a different time and place since the nature of the diseases may be different.[3]　Having practiced Chinese medicine both in China and in America, I feel confident in saying that Americans do not get sick in the same way as Chinese and cannot be treated in the same way either. It is my experience that American patients suffer from considerably more stress than do average Chinese and that without fundamental lifestyle modification American patients can not achieve the full potential of acupuncture and Chinese herbal medicine.

In China, stress is, in my opinion, relatively episodic. Here in the United States, stress is endemic, continuous, and unrelieved. Often, in fact, patients and practitioners alike do not even recognize the pervasive stressors which effect their health and wellbeing. I have discussed many of these in "The Tale of the Red Tipped Tongue".[4] Here, let me just mention a few of the stressful choices and decisions most of my patients continuously have to make: where to live, with whom, for how long, with what committments, and why; what to do professionally; with whom to have sex, when, and how; whether or not to have children, when, how many, and why; what to eat and wear and why; what to do for recreation; and what kind of healthcare to seek, when, and why. Members of our society have a great deal of personal freedom but this freedom is very stressful since it requires that we decide everything for ourselves. Nothing is assumed and we lack strong, enduring social institutions. Most of the above mentioned decisions are not personal choices for Chinese.

Therefore, it is my opinion that the American practitioner of Oriental medicine must place more emphasis on lifestyle modifications and counselling than his or her contemporary Asian counterpart. We should not assume that because acupuncture protocols exist in Chinese books for certain named diseases that application of these is all that is necessary to restore health in our patients. The necessity of lifestyle counselling is especially important in the treatment of Qi and Blood diseases. The Qi creates, moves, and holds the Blood, and the Qi and *Yi* (or mind) are essentially identical.[5] Qi is function or movement and *Yi* is awareness of that function or movement. The nature of the mind and or reality itself is nothing but ceaseless movement *cum* awareness. In my experience, most of the chronic problems to which Americans are prone begin as Qi disorders. This is even more the case in gynecological problems in American women between the ages of twenty and forty and I have written elsewhere on the effects of stress as an etiology in cervical dysplasia[6], pelvic inflammatory disease[7], and premenstrual syndrome[8]. In *Bai Ling Fu Ke*, a basic Traditional Chinese Medicine manual on the cause, diagnosis, and treatment of gynecological disorders, the author, Han Bai-ling, gives seven pieces of advice for preventive care *vis a vis* menstruation.[9] It is my belief that the counselling of American patients in just such lifestyle modifications is a necessary part of truly comprehensive and successful treatment plans which not only address current symptomology but are preventive as well.

In his discussion of menstruation, Han Bai-ling begins by stating that menstruation is a normal physiological process. His first piece of advice is to avoid fear or anger and excessive emotions in general. According to Han Bai-ling, these may cause hemoptysis, menorrhagia, and leukorrhea. In other words, due to unrestraint of the Seven Passions the Blood and Fluids may flow out of their paths. Energetically this is due to a disturbance in the flow of Qi which propels the Blood and Fluids, but the reader should remember that fundamentally there is no dichotomy between Qi and emotions. Anger "makes" the Qi flow rebelliously up. Fear "allows" the Qi to flow recklessly down. This is Han Bai-ling's number one piece of advice and is, perhaps, the number one thing all of us Americans, men and women alike, need to hear. Our culture encourages us to let our emotions run wild and this, in turn, causes our Qi and Blood to run wild too. Chinese patients may be too restrained, but Americans need more restraint. Restraint is not necessarily the same as repression. Emotions may be allowed to surface within our consciousness without our being compelled to act on them. Daily deep relaxation for a least twenty minutes per day is, in my opinion, *the single most important therapy* any of us who suffer from Qi disturbances can do. Without calming the disturbed mind, acupuncture and herbs to regulate the Qi will only be marginally effective and will not achieve long term, lasting results. Likewise our patients should be advised not to indulge themselves in too much music, tv, movies, reading, and entertainment in general which might cause elevated background levels of emotional excitement.

Han Bai-ling's second piece of advice is to avoid excessive fatigue prior to or during menstruation so as to prevent damage to the *Chong* and *Ren*. The *Chong Mai* and *Ren Mai* are two of the Eight Extraordinary or Ancestral meridians. The two channels regulate the menstruation. Damage to the *Chong* and *Ren* due to fatigue or exhaustion may cause menorrhagia, leukorrhea, and uterine prolapse. When due to fatigue these are respectively diagnosed as Qi not holding the Blood menorrhagia, Kidney Qi not holding the Fluids leukorrhea, and Qi not holding up the Center uterine prolapse. In our society, most women do not do heavy physical labor. However, rushing around all day trying to manage career, relationships, family, and all the little details of our complex lifestyle can lead to exhaustion just as surely as carrying water buckets or hoeing a field. Often it is not possible to achieve a successful cure if the patient refuses to modify her lifestyle. I have one patient who is a flight attendant who has not menstruated in ten years and who will not and cannot return to health as long as she insists on flying for a living. Besides upsetting one's biological clock, flying is extremely fatiguing to the Heart and Kidneys. Activity, whether mental, physical, emotional, or sexual must be regulated by adequate rest. Rest is as essential to health and wellbeing as are food, shelter, exercise, love, and sleep.

Third, Han Bai-ling suggests that women should not dwell on negative thoughts or their frustrations. These can cause Qi Congestion which will eventually lead to Blood Stagnation. Qi Congestion and Blood Congestion may in turn create prolonged bleeding, dysmenorrhea, and amenorrhea. In our modern Western society, women are caught between a number of irreconcilable goals such as motherhood versus a career, and sexual freedom versus familial commitment. In addition, the recognition of male-dominant injustice, which has given rise to Feminism, has also instilled in many American women a pervasive sense of frustration and anger. These are difficult and complex issues. However, each woman, for her own health and wellbeing, should let go of such feelings and emotions as much as possible. Again, that is not to say that she should repress or invalidate them. Rather, she should do what she can to ameliorate her situation and relax in the face of what she alone cannot change.

Fourth, Han Bai-ling suggests that women should avoid eating cold and raw food prior to or during their periods and also that they should take care not to catch an External Cold pathogen. As he says, this will prevent the Blood from being congealed by the Cold which in turn can cause dysmenorrhea, amenorrhea, and congelated lumps in the lower abdomen. Cold restricts and retards the flow of Blood and tends to promote Stagnation. Such Stagnation can be due either to ingestion of cold foods and drinks or the invasion of Cold from the outside environment. I have, in fact, treated two women for incapacitating menstrual cramps due to their having eaten ice cream the night before their periods. In our centrally heated homes and thanks to our material wealth providing warm clothing, External Invasion of Cold induced gynecological problems are not all that common among American women.

This is in contradistinction to northern China where, according to Dr. Tao Hsi-yu, the majority of amenorrhea and dysmenorrhea is due to Cold. However, the prevalence of ice cream, cold drinks, raw salads, and other refrigerated or frozen food does contribute to and aggravate many American women's menstrual ailments.

Fifth, Han Bai-ling suggests that women should avoid having sex during their periods. According to him, sex during the period also damages athe *Chong* and *Ren* and can lead to uterine bleeding, leukorrhea, dysmenorrhea, amenorrhea, and congealed lumps in the lower abdomen. Although there are number of possible *Zheng* or patterns of disharmony for each of these named disorders, my assumption is that sex during menstruation causes Stagnant Blood. The flow of energy at this point in the cycle should be down and out and sex causes the enrgy to flow back up and in. This leads to impeded flow and incomplete discharge. This deduction is corroborated by Tibetan medicine which believes that sex during menstruation may cause uterine neoplasms.[10] Some Western gynecologists advise women with dysmenorrhea to have sex during the menses, apparently on the assumption that it will excite an improved blood flow in the pelvis. This is true in part but is incomplete from the Oriental point of view. Here, the issue is not only getting the Qi and Blood to flow but also to flow in the right direction. Many women report increased sexual desire during their menses but Oriental medicine does not believe this desire is healthy or should be indulged. In our society we have come to believe in the value of immediate gratification of all our desires but this belief is, I believe, extremely deleterious to both our individual and societal spiritual, emotional, and physical wellbeing.

Han Bai-ling's sixth piece of advice is to avoid strong, vigorous movements or exercise during menstruation so as to prevent Qi and Blood from leaving their path. Such erratic Qi flow may result in menorrhagia, hemoptysis, epistaxis and uterine bleeding. With the popularity of aerobic exercise these days, this is a timely reminder. It seems to me that many American women over-exercise in a frantic effort to maintain an adolescent figure. Often women who over-exercise suffer from psychoemotional anxiety and frustration they attempt to deal with on a somatic level. However, no amount of exercise can solve the basic human, existential dilemma that aging implies. We all need adequate exercise to maintain health, but too much exercise is neurotic.

Seventh and finally, Han Bai-ling counsels women to eat and drink moderately, to maintain regular waking and sleeping hours, to avoid eating stimulating foods, and to try to be happy in order to prevent the occurrence of *all* gynecological problems. In other words, it is Han Bai-ling's opinion that almost all gynecological problems can be prevented *if* the patient maintains mental, emotional, physical, and dietary equilibrium. Eating and drinking moderately means not eating too little or too much as in anorexia and bulimia. Avoiding stimulating foods means avoiding coffee, alcohol, sugar, chocolate, spicy, hot pungent goods, and so-called recreational drugs. Maintaining regular hours implies a well-regulated lifestyle in general with adequate exercise and rest. One's daily schedule should be in harmony with the larger macrocosmic cycles of day and night, the phases of the moon, and the seasons of the year. Trying to be happy means cultivating a positive attitude which emphasizes the good in life, in others, and in oneself. One can consciously cultivate joy, humor, and happiness which in turn promote the free and easy flow of Qi and Blood. In my experience, this seventh and summary advice of Han Bai-ling's is not only the recipe for the prevention of gynecological diseases but of almost all diseases as well and echoes Qi Bo's advice to the Yellow Emperor in the first chapter of the *Su Wen*.[11]

As I practice so-called Chinese medicine here in America, I come more and more to the conclusion that the success of acupuncture and herbal therapy is limited by our unrestrained, unbalanced lifestyles. The more we as practitioners learn to understand and stresses in our patients' lives, the more we will be able to errect realistic treatment plans with realistic goals and expectations. If patients are unwilling or unable to make necessary lifestyle modifications, no matter how major, they should be apprised without hesitation of their responsibility for their own condition. I am reminded of a Tibetan patient in *The Way Of The White Clouds* who was told that the ultimate condition for his recovery from a life-threatening disease was his becoming a monk.[12] This was an extreme and uncommon modification but sometimes life demands hard choices.

Chinese medicine is based on the assumption of cosmic or natural law. Living in violation of that law in an individualistic and hedonistic way, we array the forces of nature against us. Herbs and acupuncture are not nor should they even attempt to be substitutes for right living. Just before sitting down to type this essay a female patient of mine called to say that the herbal formula I have her had cleared up her vaginitis which only returns if she allows herself to get too stressed. On the one hand, some practitioners might simply increase the dosage of the formula, but I, on the other hand, feel it is of paramount importance that the patient learn to calm down her over-heated mind and life. In this way both her disorder and her treatment can be seen as a life's teaching rather than as an affliction, and, rather than detracting from her life, both disorder and treatment ennoble it.

That does not mean that professional practitioners should blame their patients for shortcomings in their own knowledge and intervention. It does mean, however, emphasizing the patient's responsibility for their own mental and emotional balance, diet, exercise, rest, and positive outlook on life. As the circle turns, the doctor must once again become the Sage who teaches his or her fellow friends how to regulate their lives. This can not be done in twenty minutes nor if the practitioner is running from treatment cubicle to cubicle. It also will not work if practitioners themselves are not practitioners of what they preach. If our patients are to listen seriously to our suggestions, we must be living examples of the path we set before them. In Mahayana Buddhism there are four requirements for attracting disciples, in Tibetan called the *Du-ngo Zhi*. The first three are charity, gentle speech, and encouraging others to act according to the meaning of the Dharma or the Tao. The fourth is for oneself to likewise practice according to that same meaning.[13]

ENDNOTES

1   Anon. Committee, Shanghai Coll. of TCM, *Acupuncture: A Comprehensive Text*, John O'Connor & Dan Bensky, trans. & ed. (Eastland Press), Chicago, 1981

2   Anon. Committee, Beijing, Shanghai, & Nanjing Coll. of TCM, *Essential of Chinese Acupuncture*, (Foreign Language Press), Beijing, 1980

3   Huang, et.al., *Common Terms of Traditional Chinese Medicine In English*, (Beijing Medical College), Beijing, 1980, p. 433

4   Flaws, Bob, "The Tale of the Red-tipped Tongue", *Timing & The Times*, (Blue Poppy Press), Boulder, 1985

5   Shu Chi, "Revealing the Mystery of Life", *The Wonders of QiGong*, compiled by China Sports Magazine, (Wayfarer Publications), LA, 1985, p. 17

6   Flaws, Bob, "Cervical Dysplasia: Its Diagnosis & Treatment According to Traditional Chinese Medicine", *Journal of the American Coll. of TCM*, San Francisco, #4, 1985

7   Flaws, Bob, "Pelvic Inflammatory Disease (PID): Its Differential Diagnosis & Treatment According to Traditional Chinese Medicine", *Journal of the Amer. Coll. of TCM*, SF, #3, 1985, p. 65-79

8   Flaws, Bob, "Premenstrual Syndrome (PMS): Its Differential Diagnosis & Treatment", *American Journal of Acupuncture*, Felton, CA, Vol. 13, #3, Spet, 1985

9   Han Bai-ling, *Bai Ling Fu Ke*, (Heilongjiang Peoples Press), Haerbin, 1983, p. 10.

10   Yeshe Donden, lecture notes, Boulder, Summer, 1982

11   *Nei Jing Su Wen*, Chapter One. The best translation of this section I have seen is by Paul Unschuld, *Medicine In China: A History of Ideas*, (Univ. of CA Press), Berkeley, etc., 1985, p. 277

12   Govinda, Anagorika, *The Way of the White Clouds*, (Shambala Publications), Berkeley, 1970, p. 190-1

13   Thondup, Tulku, *The Dzogchen Innermost Essence Preliminary Practice*, (Library of Tibetan Works & Archives), Dharamsala, India, 1982, p. 84-5

LEUKORRHEA & VAGINITIS

In Traditional Chinese Medicine (TCM)[1] there are fourteen major recognized gynecological disorders.[2] These are: irregular menstruation, amenorrhea, dysmenorrhea, infertility, premenstrual tension, abnormal uterine bleeding, leukorrhea, menopausal symptoms, uterine prolapse, morning sickness, malposition of the fetus, threatened miscarriage, prolonged gestation and/or prolonged or painful labor, and insufficient lactation.[3] The American practitioner may be perplexed not to find among this list vaginitis or vulvar pruritus which are common complaints in American female patients. According to Jeremy Ross, vaginitis is included under the heading of leukorrhea in Traditional Chinese Medicine along with cervicitis, endometritis, and infection of the pelvic organs.[4] This system of classification is not entirely satisfactory since it is possible to encounter vaginitis or vulvar pruritus without abnormal vaginal discharge. Below is a discussion of the major *Zheng* or patterns of disharmony Chinese medicine believes are responsible for leukorrhea and vaginitis accompanied by suggested treatments including both acupuncture and Chinese herbs.

In Chinese, *Dai Xia* is a collective term for gynecological disease in general. It also specifically refers to the "thready mucoid discharges of the vagina".[5] *Chinese-English Terminology of Traditional Chinese Medicine* distinguishes seven types of abnormal *Dai* or vaginal discharge identified by color. *Bai Dai* is an excessive white mucoid similar to egg white. *Chi Dai* is a red, thready discharge. *Chi Bai Dai*, white and red discharge, is a blood-tinged white and thready discharge. *Qing Dai* is a greenish-blue, foul vaginal discharge. *Huang Dai* is a yellowish, thready, mucoid discharge. *Hei Dai* is a "black", thready, mucoid discharge which smells like rotten fish. And *Wu Se Dai* is a variegated discharge of various colors which also smells bad. In addition, *Bai Yin* refers to a copious, white discharge from the vagina which is the female counterpart to spermatorrhea.[6]

In general, *Dai Xia*, "discharge down", is due to imbalances within the *Ren Mai* and *Dai Mai*, two of the Eight Extra or Ancestral meridians.[7] However, each of these eight different types of vaginal discharge are due to a different Chinese disease mechanisms. Unfortunately, *Chinese-English Terminology of Traditional Chinese Medicine* does not give the disease mechanisms responsible for each of these different types of *Dai*. Jeremy Ross, based on lecture notes from the Nanjing College of Traditional Chinese Medicine, distinguishes two main patterns of leukorrhea. These are dysfunction of the *Chong* and *Ren* with weakness of the *Dai Mai* due to 1) Qi and Blood Deficiency and 2) Damp Heat Seeping Downward.[8] Mr. Ross says that in both cases there may be low back pain, dizziness, and fatigue. In the first case, the discharge will be thin and white or possibly yellowish and there may be odor. In the second case, the discharge will be deep yellow and may even be tinged with blood and there may be a fetid odor. These may be accompanied by palpitations and dryness of the mouth.

C.S. Cheung and Mary Curry divide *Dai Xia* or leukorrhea into three *Zheng*. These are insufficiency of the Kidney Qi and Depletion of the Lower *Yuan* Qi, Spleen Deficiency and Liver Qi Congestion with Damp Heat Seeping Downward, and Contraction of External Damp Heat or Wet Toxin.[9] The main difference between Mr. Ross' differentiation and Dr. Cheung

94

and Ms. Curry's is that Mr. Ross lumps both Spleen Deficiency and Kidney Deficiency together and also Internal and External Damp Heat.

According to Cheung and Curry, Kidney Deficiency *Dai Xia* is caused by the Kidney Qi having lost its ability to hold or consolidate. This results in a copious dilute, clear white vaginal discharge. This may be accompanied by facial pallor, thin loose stools, clear, copious urine, low back pain, weak knees, a cold, dragging pain in the lower abdomen, a pale tongue, and bilateral sunken and thready pulses at the Foot or *Chi* position. This is primarily a Kidney Yang Deficiency resulting in the *Dai Mai*'s losing its restraining power and the *Ren Mai* losing its ability to consolidate. The *Qi Hua* function is unable to transform the Fluids and these flow down and out at leukorrhea. My assumption is that this type of leukorrhea is equivalent to *Bai Yin* mentioned above.

Spleen Deficiency with Liver Qi Congestion and Damp Heat Seeping Down actually can be divided into four separate patterns or types of leukorrhea depending upon the relative amounts of Spleen Deficiency, Liver Congestion, Dampness, and Heat. Cheung and Curry emphasize the dysfunction of the Spleen due to dietary imbalance disrupting its *Yun Hua* function. The resulting Dampness that is generated they say damages the Liver. However, in American patients I believe that, due to stress, the Liver Qi component is typically independently and psychoemotionally generated and is, in fact, the predominant factor. This can be aggravated by diet but it is usually not caused by diet. Because the Liver and Spleen share a close mutual relationship, traditionally described by the *Ke* or Control cycle or Five Phase energetics, Liver Excess tends to produce Spleen Deficiency, and Spleen Deficiency tends to allow Liver Excess. Therefore, in treating leukorrhea due to Spleen Deficiency and Liver Congestion, one must assess the relative proportions of Excess and Deficiency in determining the Root and must adjust the treatment plan accordingly.

Since the Spleen is one of the three Organs involved in the transformation and transportation of Fluids, Spleen Deficiency, if aggravated by dietary excess, often results in the Internal generation of Dampness. Since Dampness is heavy and tends to descend, it seeps from the Middle to the Lower *Jiao* or Burner. Liver Qi Congestion likewise tends to transform into Heat due to Liu Wan-su's theory of Similar Transformation. When this Heat becomes associated with the Internally generated Dampness it produces Damp Heat. Therefore, in treating Internally generated Damp Heat in the Lower Burner manifesting as leukorrhea, one must assess whether Heat or Dampness is predominant and again adjust the treatment accordingly.

Lesson 31 of *Modern and Traditional Acupuncture*, published by the Occidental Institute of Chinese Studies, makes this distinction in their breakdown of the *Zheng* responsible for leukorrhea.[10] The authors, who are anonymous, give five *Zheng* for leukorrhea. The first is Spleen Qi Deficiency. Its symptoms are a whitish discharge like saliva without odor. There are no pains either in the lower abdomen or the lumbar region. There is facial pallor, fatigue, cold hands and feet, a tendency to soft stools, and clear, copious urine. The tongue in this uncomplicated pattern is pale with a white coating and the pulse is listed as delayed and weak. These symptoms predominate in cases where Spleen Deficiency is the main or over-riding issue. However, in my experience with American patients, most have at least some Liver Qi Congestion signs and symptoms and therefore I can never remember seeing such an uncomplicated case of leukorrhea.

Under the heading Congestion of the Liver the following signs and symptoms are given: pale red or white, thickish discharge of indeterminate duration accompanied by menstrual irregularity, chest distress, depression, irritability, dry throat, a bitter taste in the mouth, a yellowish facial complexion, normal stools, yellow urine, a yellowish white coating on the tongue, and a wiry pulse.

Actually, here we should distinguish between simple Liver Qi Congestion signs and symptoms and Depressive Liver Heat signs and symptoms. If there is a reddish discharge it would point to Heat as opposed to simple Qi Congestion and would be accompanied by the bitter mouth, irritability, and yellow tongue fur; the urine would not necessarily be yellow; and the throat might not be dry since these would indicate only Qi Congestion without the presence of Heat. The pulse would be wiry in either case but the tip of the tongue would be redder the more Heat there is.

Heat tends to be Excess in the week preceding menstruation due to the growth of Yang[11] and this is when the Liver also becomes most Congested. Therefore, signs and symptoms due to Qi Congestion and Congestive Heat often manifest during this phase of the cycle. It is also common for Qi Congestion to transform into Heat during this phase. In either case the stools may not, in fact, be normal. Typically Qi Congestion causes constipation. The thick consistency of this discharge is usually identified as a yeast infection by Western gynecology. As implied by Cheung and Curry and according to my experience, these two *Zheng*, Spleen Deficiency and Liver Congestion are most commonly met with in tandem.

The third *Zheng* the OICS authors describe is listed as Phlegm Dampness. The discharge is described as abundant and like "glairy" mucous. This type of leukorrhea is encountered in obese women. It is accompanied by fatigue, a heavy head, a tasteless mouth, chest oppression, abdominal swelling or lumps, abundant phlegm production, small appetite, strong and rapid respiration, a greasy moist coating on the tongue, and a slippery pulse. This is an idealized picture which in the clinic may be complicated by either or both Liver Qi or Spleen Deficiency.

OICS' last two *Zheng* are Humidity Heat (or Damp Heat) and Insufficiency of the Kidneys. We have discussed Insufficiency of the Kidneys above and the OICS' description does not offer any new or different information. In terms of Damp Heat, it is not completely clear to me whether the OICS authors are describing specifically External Damp Heat or if, like Mr. Ross, they have lumped both External and Internal Damp Heat together under the assumption that their treatment would be the same in any case. The symptoms given for Damp Heat leukorrhea are an abundant, thick, yellow discharge at times tinged with blood with slightly strong odor, fatigue, a heavy head, thirst but no desire to drink, anxiety and restlessness, abnormal stools, disturbed sleep, red urine, possible urethritis, a moist, yellow coated tongue, and a superficial, small, and rapid pulse. The superficial pulse would seem to point to an External pathogen.

Vaginitis as a symptom may or may not be accompanied by leukorrhea. In my experience, vaginitis or vulvar pruritus may accompany Spleen Qi Deficiency with Liver Congestion turning to Heat and Internally and Externally generated Damp Heat in the Lower *Jiao*. However, there is another disease mechanism which we have not mentioned which may also cause vaginitis without *Dai Xia* or leukorrhea. This is Kidney Yin Deficiency with Deficient Fire in the Lower Burner. Its symptoms are a dry vaginal irritation without discharge, fatigue, anxiety or restlessness, possible night sweats, palpitations, insomnia, tinnitus, low back pain, sore knees, post meridianal malar flushing or tidal fever, scant menstrual discharge, nocturia, bleeding gums without pain, a tender, red-tipped, apically fluted or red, cracked tongue with scant, slightly yellow fur, and a thready, fastish pulse with a deep left *Chi* position. The patient may complain of dry skin in general and is often thin as opposed to being heavy-set. Typically the irritation will manifest or become aggravated after the period when the Blood in the *Chong Mai* is weak[12] which in turn weakens the body's systemic Yin. This type of vaginitis is also seen in women who have had complete hysterectomies and who are not on hormone replacement therapy. In addition, I have encountered this *Zheng* in women who have chronic, post-period herpes genitalia outbreaks. This pattern of disharmony is aggravated by stress, fatigue, excess sex, sugar, alcohol, and recreational drugs. It is usually a deep-seated, chronic pattern recalcitrant to treatment.

Herpes genitalia is a kind of vaginitis. In my experience it can begin as either External Invasion of Damp Heat or as Internally generated Damp Heat due to Depressive Liver Fire and Spleen Deficiency. Often this is even further complicated by simultaneous or eventual Kidney Yin Deficiency with Deficient Fire in the Lower Burner. The relationship between the Liver, Spleen, Kidneys, and Deficiency Fire has been described by me in some detail in "The Tale of the Red-tipped Tongue".[13] There are numerous combinations this complicated scenario can have and correctly identifying all the factors and assigning them their proper importance in a treatment plan is often difficult and attended by much trial and error. In herpes genitalia, it is also necessary that the concept of *Du* or Toxins must also be taken into account when treating herbally.

I have said that herpes genitalia can be either Externally or Internally generated. Typically the first outbreak is an External Invasion. However, subsequent outbreaks are usually due to diet, stress, menstrual cycle, fatigue, and sex and have to do primarily with the Internal metabolism. I have seen two cases of herpes genitalia diagnosed by Western MDs which were not transmitted sexually, one in a ten year old girl who

99

was not yet sexually active. This leads me to believe that herpes genitalia can be generated by entirely Internal imbalances involving Liver, Spleen, and Kidneys. It is difficult to talk about curing herpes genitalia. Patients can go for years without an occurrence and then, due to an infelicitous combination of stress, fatigue, diet, etc., have an outbreak. However, Chinese medicine can, in my experience, significantly reduce its frequency, virulence, and recuperation time.

In the last couple of years, candidiasis or yeast infection has been advanced as the latest theory for the causation of many chronic symptoms in otherwise "undiagnosable" patients, and a yeast-free diet has been touted as the current panacea. Although in many patients such a diet can help to drastically reduce their symptomology, I do not think this theory of disease causation is ultimately very sophisticated. Since yeast infections in the vaginal tract are commonly encountered in clinical practice here in America, a few words on this subject seem germane.

Patients diagnosed as being systemically yeast intolerant are put on a very restrictive, yeast-free diet. Depending upon the severity of their symptoms, they may also be given nystatin. Nystatin is an antifungal, antimycotic antibiotic. Nystatin attacks and breaks down the cell walls of fungi and yeast thus killing them. By avoiding all foods which may be contaminated with yeast, the patient may reduce the symptoms caused by yeast infection. However, as far as I can tell, if the patient eats yeast-contaminated foods even after having hewed to the diet for an extended period of time, their symptoms will return. In other words, a strict, yeast-free diet does not seem to alter the body's metabolism in a fundamental way which over time eliminates the body's intolerance. Likewise, although nystatin is not listed as having any side-effects, complications, or restriction, it also does not fundamentally alter the patient's physiology in such a way so as to restore balance and harmonious function. Truly healthy people are not allergic to yeast.

Some of the foods which are the most aggravating to people diagnosed as suffering from candidiasis can be explained from a Chinese energetic point of view. For instance, wine is usually very aggravating for patients with candidiasis. Wine is sour-tasting and therefore "enters" the Liver. Alcohol produces both Dampness and Heat internally. While it tends to make the Stomach Hot, it simultaneously tends to make the Spleen Damp. Patients whose Chinese diagnosis is Liver Qi Congestion and Spleen Deficiency with Damp Heat in the Lower Burner who also present so-called yeast-induced symptoms will typically find their symptoms aggravated by the ingestion of alcohol in general and wine in particular. Avoiding wine is a part of a comprehensive Chinese treatment plan for this scenario, but that alone is not enough to restore the patient's balance. Relaxation, exercise, diet, herbs, and acupuncture may all be used to restore the body's functional harmony. Once that balance is restored, the patient should be able to eat and drink a moderate amount of yeast-contaminated foods and beverages without experiencing ill effect.

Both leukorrhea and vaginitis can be treated by either acupuncture or Chinese herbs or a combination of the two. In terms of acupuncture, both Jeremy Ross[16] and the authors of OICS[17] agree that, no matter what the pattern of disharmony, one can base the erection of an acupuncture treatment plan on a foundation of three points: *Dai Mai* (GB 26), *San Yin Jiao* (Sp 6), and *Qi Hai (CV 6)*. *Dai Mai* regulates the *Dai Mai*, *Ren Mai*, and *Chong Mai* and is also the crossing point of the *Dai Mai* and the Foot *Shao Yàng*. It is a specific experience point for the treatment of *Dai Xia*. *San Yin Jiao* regulates the Three Yin of the leg, circulates the pelvis, and catalyzes both the Spleen and Kidneys to transform and transport Fluids. *Qi*

101

Hai regulates both the *Ren Mai* and the *Chong Mai* and catalyzes the Qi to again transform and transport Fluids. Then, depending upon the specific *Zheng*, one can add appropriate points to tailor the treatment. Without such customization, the therapeutic results will be less than satisfactory.

For Spleen Qi Deficiency one can add *Zu San Li* (St 36) and *Pi Shu* (Bl 20). For Spleen Yang Deficiency these points plus *Zhong Wan* (CV12) can be moxaed indirectly with either *Fu Zi* cakes[18] or *Tai Yi* Moxa rolls[19]. For Damp Spleen, *Shang Qiu* (Sp 5) and *Yang Ling Quan* (GB 34) can be added. For Phlegm Dampness, needle *Feng Long* (St 40), *Zu San Li*, and *Zhong Wan.* For Liver Qi Congestion, needle *Tai Chong* (Liv 3) and *Li Gou* (Liv 5). *Li Gou* is the *Luo* point of the Foot *Jue Yin*, and the longitudinal *Luo* of the Liver encircles the genitalia. If there is Liver Fire producing pronounced inflammation, one can choose instead Foot *Zhong Du* (Liv 6), the *Xi* cleft point of the Foot *Jue Yin, Qu Quan* (Liv 8), its *He* Sea point, and *Xing Jian* (Liv 2). *Zhong Du* is useful for relieving acute pain and congestion on the Liver meridian and *Qu Quan* spreads Stagnant Liver Qi, dispels Damp Heat, and clears the Lower *Jiao. Xing Jian* is the dispersal point of the Liver and reduces Liver Fire. For Kidney Yang Deficiency, moxa *Shen Shu* (Bl 23), *Ming Men* (GV 4), and *Guan Yuan* (CV 4) and use *Bu Fa* (tonification technique) on the three main points. For Damp Heat, use *Zhong Ji* (CV 3), *Yin Ling Quan* (Sp 9), and *Xue Hai* (Sp 10) if it is External Damp Heat. If it is Internal Damp Heat, use *Zhong Ji, Yin Ling Quan, Xing Jian,* and *Li Gou. Zhong Ji* is a local point which regulates the Lower *Jiao* to eliminate Damp Heat. When used with *Li Gou* it eliminates specifically Liver Fire from the Lower *Jiao.* For Damp Heat leukorrhea/vaginitis, use strong reducing technique (*Xie Fa*) and retain the needles for up to one hour. Treat daily or even twice per day until the symptoms' virulence diminishes. For Yin Deficiency vulvar

102

pruritus, needle with *Bu Fa San Yin Jiao, Tai Xi* (Ki 3), *Tai Chong, Yin Gu* (Ki 10), and *Heng Gu* (Ki 11). *San Yin Jiao* strengthens the Three Yin of the leg. *Tai Xi* and *Tai Chong* are the *Yuan* Source points of the Kidneys and Liver. The Kidneys are the Root of Yin and the Liver stores the Blood. Therefore they share a close mutual relationship vis a vis the Yin. The *Yuan* points are used to balance the Yin and Yang within their respective organs. *Yin Gu* is the Water point of the Kidneys and *Heng Gu* is a local point for treatment of pain in the genitalia. *Heng Gu* is located on the Foot *Shao Yin* and is believed by some people to connect with the *Chong Mai*.[20]

There are a number of Chinese herbal formulae useful in the treatment of leukorrhea and vaginitis. These can also be schematized according to the differentiation of *Zheng*. Long Dan Xie Gan Tang (Dragon Gall Disperse the Liver Decoction) is perhaps the most often thought of Chinese formula for vaginitis and other inflammations of the pelvis. Its ingredients are:

> Radix Gentianae
> Radix Scutellariae
> Fructus Gardeniae
> Rhizoma Alismatis
> Semen Plantaginis
> Caulis Akebiae Mu Tong
> Radix Rehmanniae
> Apex Radicis Angelicae Sinensis
> Radix Bupleuri
> Radix Glycyrrhizae

This formula is for either Liver Fire leukorrhea and vaginitis and/or Damp Heat in the Lower *Jiao*. It should only be used with relatively strong patients and even then for only a few days. Its ingredients are very Cold and dispersing. If the patient's condition is subacute and their constitution is

103

weak,this formula will not achieve the desired results and may make the condition even more recalcitrant and complicated. As the inflammation and signs of Heat abate, the patient should be switched to a more moderate formula which both attacks the Evil and supports the Righteous. This formula is heavily weighted towards attacking and dispersing.

Da Huang Mu Dan Pi Tang (Rhubarb and Moutan Decoction) is also for a strong patient with Excess Heat in the Lower *Jiao*. In this case Heat is predominant and Dampness is nonexistent or minor. This Heat is generated by or involved with Blood Stagnation. The patient may have lumps or pain with pressure in the lower abdomen. In addition, they should be constipated before choosing this formula. The tongue coating is yellow and dry and the pulse is slow and tight. The patient may also have a history of dysmenorrhea, amenorrhea, and/or clots in their menstrual discharge. The ingredients in this formula are:

> Rhizoma Rhei
> Cortex Radicis Moutan
> Semen Persicae
> Semen Benincasae
> Mirabilitum

Ba Wei Dai Xia Fang (Eight Ingredient Formula for Leukorrhea) is a more moderate formula. It is for Damp Heat in the Lower *Jiao* in a patient of moderate to strong confirmation whose inflammation is subacute. Its ingredients are:

> Radix Angelicae Sinensis
> Radix Ligustici Wallichi
> Sclerotium Poriae Cocoris
> Pericarpium Viridis Citri Reticulatae
> Caulis Akebiae Mu Tong
> Cortex Smilacis Glabrae

104

Flos Lonicerae
Rhizoma Rhei

This formula is primarily for External Damp Heat which has become entrenched due to Deficient Blood and poor circulation in the pelvis. The Rhubarb can be adjusted or omitted depending upon the presence or absence of constipation and the state of the patient's Righteous Qi.

Dan Zhi Xiao Yao Tang (Free and Easy Decoction with Moutan and Gardenia) is for moderate to weak patients with Liver Qi Congestion turning to Fire and Spleen and Blood Deficiency. This is a very useful formula for treating American females. It can be modified in many ways to fit the presenting situation. Its ingredients are:

Radix Bupleuri
Radix Angelicae Sinensis
Radix Paeoniae Albae
Rhizoma Atractylodis Macrocephalae
Sclerotium Poriae Cocoris
Cortex Radicis Moutan
Fructus Gardeniae
Radix Praeparatus Glycyrrhizae

To make this formula more specifically effective for Damp Heat leukorrhea and vaginitis, Radix Sophorae, Phellodendron, Fructus Cnidii, Semen Euryalis, and/or Semen Gingko may be added. If there is simultaneous Yin Deficiency, Artemesia Capillaris may be substituted for Bupleurum and Yin tonic herbs such as Eclipta, Dendrobium, and Ligustrum Lucidum can be added. Likewise, Codonopsis and Astragalus can be added to further strengthen the Spleen and Qi and Persica and Salvia Miltorrhiza can be added to address Blood Stagnation.

Wan Dai Tang (Decoction to End Leukorrhea) is, in fact,

similar to Xiao Yao Tang. However, in this formula the emphasis is on Spleen Deficiency and Dampness with less attention being paid to Liver Qi and Heat. Its ingredients are:

> Rhizoma Atractylodis Macrocephalae
> Rhizoma Praeparata Atractylodis
> Radix Dioscoreae
> Radix Codonopsis Pilosulae
> Radix Paeoniae Albae
> Semen Plantaginis
> Pericarpium Citri Reticulatae
> Flos Seu Herba Carbonisata Schizonepetae
> Radix Bupleuri
> Radix Glycyrrhizae

Atractylodes Macrocephela, Rhizoma Atractylodis, Dioscorea, and Codonopsis tonify the Spleen and rid Dampness. Pericarpium Citri Reticulatae descends the Turbid and Semen Plantaginis promotes the seeping of Dampness through urination. Peony relaxes the Liver and tonifies the Blood, while small doses of Bupleurum and Schizonepeta address dredging the Liver as a minor issue.

Gui Fu Di Huang Wan (Cinnamon & Aconite with Rehmannia Pills) with modifications is indicated for Spleen and Kidney Yang Deficiency. Its ingredients include:

> Cortex Cinnamomi
> Radix Aconiti Carmichaeli
> Radix Rehmanniae Conquitae
> Rhizoma Alismatis
> Sclerotium Poriae Cocoris
> Radix Dioscoreae
> Semen Cuscutae
> Os Sepiae
> Fructus Psoraleae

106

Herba Artemesiae Anomelae
Flos Celosiae

The first six ingredients are also known as Jin Gui Shen Qi Wan (Golden Cabinet Kidney Qi Pills) and comprise the most famous Kidney Yang tonic formula. Cuscuta, Psoralea, and Os Sepia are added specifically to consolidate and astringe the *Jing* or Essence thus ending the leukorrhea. Interestingly, Artemesia Anomala is for ridding Stagnant Blood, and Flos Celosiae is for purging Liver Fire. This shows how typically poor pelvic circulation and Liver Entanglement complicate most cases of *Dai Xia*.

Jing Xin Lian Zi Yin (Clear the Heart Lotus Seed Drink) is also for Spleen Kidney Deficiency leukorrhea. However it is for Spleen and Kidney Qi Deficiency, not Yang Deficiency. Instead of stoking the Fire of the *Ming Men*, it purges the Fire of the Heart with Lotus Seed and Scutellaria and purges Excessive *Ming Men Huo* with Semen Plantaginis and Cortex Radicis Lycii. By dispersing the Heart, Liver Fire is likewise reduced. By tonifying the Kidney and Liver Yin with Fructus Lycii, Fire is held in check and communication between the Heart and Kidneys is restored. This formula is effective in treating nervous patients with Kidney Spleen Deficiency leukorrhea with simultaneous Deficiency Fire in the Heart. Its ingredients are:

> Semen Nelumbinis
> Radix Codonopsis Pilosulae
> Radix Astragali Seu Hedysari
> Tuber Ophiopogonis
> Sclerotium Poriae Cocoris
> Semen Plantaginis
> Cortex Radicis Lycii
> Fructus Lycii
> Radix Scutellariae

Radix Glycyrrhizae

The last formula is Zhi Bai Di Huang Wan (Anemarrhena & Phellodendron with Rehmannia Pills). This is a famous and standard formula for Flaring of Deficient Fire due to Yin Deficiency of the Kidneys. Although this formula may be used for leukorrhea it may also be used for dry vulvar pruritis and chronic genital herpes without vaginal discharge. Often this occurs after the period when the Blood and therefore the Yin are depleted. This formula may be modified by the inclusion of such Blood-tonifying herbs as Dang Gui and Fructus Lycii and by Yin-tonifying and moistening herbs such as Eclipta, Dendrobium, Ophiopogon, and Ligustrum Lucidum. This formula is contraindicated in patients with weak digestion and a tendency to diarrhea. Since Yin Deficiency results in Qi Deficiency and since the Kidney Yin is intimately connected with the Large Intestine through the Internal Gate of the Triple Heater, in many cases, the simultaneous administration of Bu Zhong Yi Qi Tang or Wan can help mitigate the sometimes "greasy" effects of this formula and protect the digestion at the same time as tonifying the Qi. The standard ingredients of Zhi Bai Di Huang Wan are:

Rhizoma Anemarrhenae
Cortex Phellodendri
Radix Rehmanniae Conquitae
Fructus Corni
Radix Dioscoreae
Rhizoma Alismatis
Cortex Radicis Moutan
Sclerotium Poriae Cocoris

If vaginal inflammation due to Damp Heat is severe, a douche can be made from the following:

Fructus Cnidii

Radix Sophorae
Fructus Meliae
Cortex Phellodendri
Cortex Radicis Lycii
Alum

This is called She Chuang Zi Chong Xi Ji (Cnidium Fruit Decoction for Vaginitis). For less severe pruritus, Mopiko Ointment applied topically is also useful. Initially it will sting on application but the net effect will be reduced itching and inflammation. Other douches, such as with boric acid, vinegar, or yogurt, are also useful based on the patient's empirical experience. For herpetic lesions in the weeping stage which are slow to scab, a topical application of powdered Realgar mixed with isopropyl alcohol will promote faster healing. It should be applied several times per day. This is not useful once the lesion has scabbed and it should be discontinued if it causes any irritation to the surrounding skin.

The selection of acupuncture and/or herbs in the treatment plan depends both on the Chinese *Bian Zheng* and the individual patient. If the practitioner has recourse to both modalities, I suggest using both acupuncture and herbs in acute and Excess cases and only herbs in chronic and Deficiency cases. One might also choose to use both herbs and acupuncture until the inflammation and pain are alleviated and then rely primarily on the herbs alone. In Kidney Yang Deficiency cases, the patient or her family can be taught how to apply moxa themselves. However, if one does not have access to Chinese herbs or the knowledge and experience to use them, acupuncture alone can treat *Dai Xia* and vaginitis. For acute and Excess cases, the treatment will be relatively brief. For chronic and Deficiency cases, the treatments may be spaced out to once or twice per week but the entire course of treatment will be relatively long.

It is Cheung and Curry's opinion that External Damp Heat or Wet Toxin should be treated by a combination of Western allopathic medicine, presumably antibiotics, and Traditional Chinese Medicine.[23] In China, such a combination is sometimes referred to as *Hong Yi* or Red Medicine and also as New Medicine.[24] Cheung and Curry do not elaborate on the details of such a treatment plan, presumably to prevent an inexperienced practitioner attempting to treat a serious and virulent infection with insufficient knowledge. They do mention that this category of *Dai Xia* covers the Western diagnoses of pelvic inflammation, suppurative endometritis, cervicitis, Trichomonas vaginitis, Candida vaginal infection, and senile vaginitis. Although one of the weak points of Chinese medicine is its inability to look directly into the body and assess the virulence of endometrial infection, still, with care and caution, I believe one can successfully treat such inflammatory disorders with Chinese medicine without necessary recourse to allopathic intervention. I have written on the diagnosis and treatment of pelvic inflammatory disease elsewhere.[25] Although resort to antibiotic therapy should not be ruled out, in my experience, aggressive herbal therapy and twice daily acupuncture treatments coupled with herbal douches can treat acute pelvic and vaginal infections.

Parenthetically, Cheung and Curry say that this *Zheng* is due to "bad healthcare (and to) residing in a wet location for a long time (which) may lead to the contraction of worm(s) and bacteria (thus) causing excessive vaginal discharge."[26] In *Bai Ling Fu Ke (Bai Ling On Gynecology)* a formula is given for the treatment of prurulent vaginitis which consists of wrapping certain herbs in a piece of raw liver which is then inserted in the vagina.[27] Han Bai-ling, the author, states that the "worms" will be attracted to the liver and will then be killed by the herbs inside. I do not think many American women would accept this kind of therapy but it is an interesting idea.

Depending upon the *Bian Zheng*, more or less attention must be paid in the treatment plan to diet and lifestyle. For cases involving marked Spleen Deficiency and Spleen Dampness, diet will be an important and indispensable part of the therapy. Such patients should be advised to avoid or minimize foods which weaken the Middle Qi and produce Dampness. This includes raw vegetables, cold or frozen foods and drinks, dairy products, sugar, and greasy foods. For cases involving Liver Qi and Liver Fire, greasy foods, alcohol, spicy, hot pungent foods, and especially coffee, both caffeinated and decaff, should be avoided or minimized. However, since Qi Congestion is primarily psychoemotionally generated, diet in such cases is not as important. For these patients, programmed relaxation and exercise and general stress reduction are relatively more important and ultimately indispensable. In cases involving weakness of the Kidneys, both Yin and/or Yang, patients are advised to avoid or minimize cold and frozen foods and drinks, sugar, salt, alcohol, coffee, and black tea. In addition, they should be very careful in matters of the bedroom. They should also be sure to eat adequate protein. In the treatment of acute cases of External Damp Heat or Wet Toxin, diet is relatively less important. Patients should avoid shrimp, lobster, and shellfish in general and should not eat too much chicken. The patient should rest as much as possible. As the inflammation subsides, however, attention to diet and lifestyle should be emphasized to prevent or deal with a chronic, deep-seated, lingering imbalance.

The following is a case history of a woman with Yin Deficiency, Deficient Heat vaginitis. I have chosen this case because this *Zheng* has not been discussed previously in any of the English language literature in relationship to vaginitis and since, as I have pointed out in "The Tale of the Red-tipped Tongue"[28], this pattern of imbalance is very common amongst Americans.

This woman was thirty-two years old. Her major complaint was non-specific vaginitis. She had tried a number of therapies before coming to me but none had been significantly helpful. The patient complained of a dry irritation and the absence of vaginal lubrication. There was a slight "gluey", pale yellow discharge. This had begun one year previous when she had had a Copper 7 IUD inserted. The Copper 7 had come out accidentally one month prior to her first visit. The discharge had abated somewhat since then but still persisted. The patient had had three IUDs over the last fifteen years. At twenty she had had PID due to a Dalkon Shield which had been treated with antibiotics. This had left severe adhesions on her tubes and ovaries. Six and a half years previous the patient had had an abortion and a D & C when three months pregnant. From menarche until the birth of her first child, the patient had had severe dysmenorrhea with nausea and also severe PMS. Her youngest child was four years old. Now she experienced some stabbing, right-sided pain in the lower abdomen and some premenstrual breast tenderness and occasional irritability. Her menstrual cycle was regular and her flow was bright red but scanty. The patient remarked that her flow was almost nothing since her last pregnancy. Her bowel movements were irregular, hard, dry, and piecemeal. Sometimes, however, her stools would begin hard and end loose and she experienced loose stools consistently before each period. Her urination was frequent and she had nocturia every night. She experienced occasional orthostatic hypotension and anxiety attacks with rapid heartbeat. In addition, she had a history of chronic bladder infections with dysuria and hematuria. She had had mononucleosis as a child and non-infectious hepatitis four years previous accompanied by emaciation, nausea, and vomiting. Her tongue was pale, thin, fluted, and tender with a red tip and a moist coating. Her pulse was extremely fine and deep with sunken and weak *Chi* positions bilaterally. In her left pulse there was also a hint of wiriness.

My diagnosis was Liver Congestion, Spleen Deficiency, and Yin Deficiency with some Stagnant Blood and Deficiency Heat and Dryness in the Lower *Jiao*. My prescription was a modified version of Hei Xiao Yao Tang (Black Free and Easy Decoction). Its ingredients were:

Radix Bupleuri	9 grams
Radix Paeoniae Albae	9 "
Radix Angelicae Sinensis	9 "
Sclerotium Poriae Cocoris	9 "
Rhizoma Atractylodis	
Macrocephalae	9 "
Radix Rehmanniae	15 "
Tuber Ophiopogonis	15 "
Radix Scrophulariae	15 "
Herba Dendrobii	15 "
Radix Salviae Miltorrhizae	9 "
Rhizoma Anemarrhenae	9 "
Cortex Phellodendri	6 "
Radix Praeparatus	
Glycyrrhizae	6 "

One *bao* or packet of the above was to be taken over a period of two days in decoction. After four *bao* of the above, the patient reported that her vaginal discharge was much better but her labia were still inflamed. She still could not wear pants. Also, she was constipated and her stomach was upset. I decided that the Yin tonic herbs were disturbing her digestion so I decided to emphasize her digestion and constipation and vaginitis. Therefore, I needled *San Yin Jiao, Zhao Hai* (Ki 6), *Zu San Li, Tian Shu* (St 25), *Yang Ling Quan*, and *Heng Gu*. The herbal formula I prescribed at this time consisted of:

Radix Bupleuri	9 grams
Radix Paeoniae Albae	6 "
Radix Angelicae Sinensis	6 "

113

Sclerotium Poriae Cocoris	9	"
Rhizoma Atractylodis		
Macrocephalae	9	"
Rhizoma Pinelliae	9	"
Pericarpium Citri		
Reticulatae	6	"
Pericarpium Viride Citri		
Reticulatae	6	"
Semen Trichosanthis	9	"
Semen Cannabis	6	"
Rhizoma Recens Zingiberis	3 slices	

After one week the patient reported a continuing tendency to constipation although she had had a number of bowel movements. There was still a tiny amount of vaginal discharge but the irritation and inflammation was almost all gone. One month later the patient again complained of minimal vaginal irritation and a chronic sore throat due to stress and overwork. Acupuncture, using Dr. Manaka's Ion Pumping Cord, immediately relieved both symptoms. A silver needle was inserted in right *Da Ling* (Per 7) and a gold needle in left *Tai Chong* to which were attached the black and red leads respectively. Three months later the patient reported having caught an intestinal flu with vomiting and diarrhea. This was followed by an acute flare-up of her vaginitis due to Fluid Dryness aggravating her underlying Yin Deficiency. My prescription at that time was:

Radix Bupleuri	9 grams	
Radix Paeoniae Albae	9	"
Rhizoma Atractylodis		
Macrocephalae	9	"
Sclerotium Poriae Cocoris	9	"
Radix Praeparatus		
Glycyrrhizae	6	"
Radix Scrophulariae	15	"

Tuber Ophiopogonis	15 "
Radix Rehmanniae	15 "
Herba Dendrobii	15 "
Rhizoma Anemarrhenae	6 "
Cortex Phellodendri	6 "

Ten *bao* over a period of twenty days eliminated the patient's vaginitis. At this time her bowel movements were normal. Unfortunately, but all too typically, the patient had recently started a new business and felt she could not rest and make her health her priority. She was content to deal with her health crises on an ad hoc basis and was not willing to follow a comprehensive treatment plan including programmed relaxation and lifestyle modifications. Therefore, I doubt very much if this will be the end of her gynecological problems.

ENDNOTES

1   Traditional Chinese Medicine or TCM is the state-approved version of Chinese medicine in the Peoples Republic of China. This is only one style of Chinese medicine. It is based on Confucianism and the *Han Xue Pai* movement of the Qing dynasty as interpreted by dialectical materialism.

2   There are a number of additional recognized obstetrical disorders in Chinese medicine which I have described in *Path Of Pregnancy*, (Paradigm Publications), Brookline MA, 1983

3   Ross, Jeremy, "Traditional Chinese Medicine and Gynecology, Part One", *The Journal Of Chinese Medicine*, UK, No. 11, Jan. 1983, p. 21

4   Ross, Jeremy, "Traditional Chinese Medicine and Gynecology, Part Two", *The Journal Of Chinese Medicine*, UK, No. 12, May 1983, p.9

5   Liao, Sung J., *Chinese-English Terminology Of Traditional Chinese Medicine*, (Hunan Science & Technology Press), 1981, p. 610

6   Ibid., p. 610-11

7   Anonymous, *Modern & Traditional Acupuncture*, "Lesson 31, A Treatment Formulary", Occidental Institute of Chinese Studies, Miami, date?, p. 131

8   Ross, op. cit., #11, p. 12

9   Cheung, C.S. & Curry, Mary, "Leukorrhea", *Journal Of The Am. Coll. Of Trad. Chin. Med.*, SF, #3, 1982, p. 41

10   OICS, op. cit., p. 131-2

11   Ross, op. cit., #11, p. 19

12   Ibid., p. 18

13   Flaws, Bob, "The Tale of the Red-tipped Tongue", *Timing And The Times*, (Blue Poppy Press), Boulder, 1986

14   Long, James, W., *The Essential Guide to Prescription Drugs*, (Harper & Row), NY, etc., 1985, p. 568

15   Jin Zi-jiu, *Jin Zi-Jiu Zhuan Ji*, trans. by Michael Helme, excerpted in *Timing And The Times*, op. cit., p. 128

16   Ross, op. cit., #12, p. 12

17   OICS, op. cit., p. 131-2

18   *Fu zi* cakes: herbal cakes about 3/8" thick and 1 1/2" in diameter comprised of powdered Aconite and other herbs bound with honey and pressed, upon which moxa is burned indirectly

19   *Tai Yi* moxa rolls include Artemesia Vulgaris and Cinnamon, Dried Ginger, Cloves, Sichuan Pepper, Realgar, Saussurea, Angelica Duhuo, Angelica Dahurica, Asarum, Atractylodes (*Cang Shu*), Myrrh, and Frankincense. They are especially effective in the treatment of Deficiency digestive disorders.

117

20   Low, Royston, *The Secondary Vessels Of Acupuncture,* (Thorsons Publishers), UK, 1983, p. 173-4

21   Bensky, Dan & Gamble, Andrew, *Chinese Herbal Medicine, Materia Medica,* (Eastland Press), Seattle, 1986, p. 413 & 88 respectively

22   Hsu Hong-yen & Hsu Chau-shin, *Commonly Used Chinese Herb Formulas With Illustrations,* (Oriental Healing Arts Institute), LA, 1980, p. 165

23   Cheung & Curry, op. cit., p. 42

24   Unschuld, Paul U., *Medicine In China, A History Of Ideas,* (U of CA Press), Berkeley, etc., 1985, p. 252-60

25   Flaws, Bob, "Pelvic Inflammatory Disease: Its Diagnosis & Treatment According to Traditional Chinese Medicine", *Journal of The Am. Coll. Of Trad. Chin. Med.,* SF, forthcoming

26   Cheung & Curry, op. cit., p. 42

27   Han Bai-ling, *Bai Ling Fu Ke,* (Heilongjiang Peoples Press), Haerbin, PRC, 1983, p. 151

28   Flaws, "The Tale of the Red-tipped Tongue", op. cit.

DYSFUNCTIONAL UTERINE BLEEDING

Dysfunctional uterine bleeding, also known as functional uterine bleeding, is a commonly encountered complaint in clinical practice. Both Western allopathic and Chinese traditional medicine have their own theories on its causation and therapies for its treatment. It is my opinion that the Chinese model and method of treatment for this disorder has much to recommend it when compared with the allopathic approach. Traditional Chinese Medicine often treats this problem successfully without recourse to such heroic measures as surgery. In addition, Chinese treatment is usually low in cost, is without iatrogenic complications, and, because it treats the whole person and not just a single, isolated symptom, it typically results in improvements in the patient's health and well-being on many levels. However, since allopathic medicine and the materialist biological science on which it is based are the dominant conceptual matrices in the West, American practitioners of Chinese medicine should also be generally familiar with the description and treatment of this disorder from the Western point of view.

According to the *Merck Manual*, dysfunctional uterine bleeding is defined as abnormal uterine bleeding not associated with neoplasm, inflammation, or pregnancy. Although it can occur at any time in a menstruant woman, adolescence and the climacteric are the most typical times for it to manifest.

According to Western biological science, dysfunctional uterine bleeding is due to hormonal imbalance -- specifically excessive or unopposed estrogen stimulation. "The estrogen may be endogenous from an estrogen-producing ovarian tumor (e.g. granulosa cell tumor), polycystic ovaries (Stein-Levanthal syndrome), or abnormal estrogen metabolism (liver disease)...".[1] Irregular or excessive estrogen ingestion, as in hormone replacement or supplementation therapy, should also be ruled out.

Allopathic treatment for dysfunctional uterine bleeding may include dilation and curettage (D & C) and/or hormone ingestion therapy. However, control of excessive bleeding will not necessarily correct the lack of ovulation and the consequent infertility which usually accompany this disorder. Estrogen-producing neoplasms are removed surgically. For patients with polycystic ovaries, ovarian wedge resection is often resorted to. For endometrial hyperplasia during the climacteric, curettage alone is effective in fifty percent of the cases. However, if repeated curettage is not successful, hysterectomy is typically advised. For carcinoma in situ, hysterectomy is likewise recommended.

From the traditional Chinese medical point of view, all these allopathic treatments have drawbacks and potential iatrogenic complications. Hormone therapy requires frequent patient examinations which are expensive. In addition, hormones are a natural Pure Essence and their lack or imbalance denotes a systemic metabolic imbalance which simple hormonal replacement or supplementation may not address systemically. In other words, the patient is not seen holistically and other complaints may not receive comprehensive treatment. These other, supposedly unrelated complaints may eventually, over time, lead to a life-threatening situation. And further, the possible adverse side-effects of estrogen are accentuation of migraine headaches, breast enlargement, congestion, and tenderness, hypertension, thrombophlebitis, pulmonary embolism, retinal embolism, coronary embolism, stroke, depression, jaundice, and increased susceptibility to yeast infections.[2]

Curettage is a local treatment which likewise does nothing to harmonize the patient's entire metabolism. It is an invasive procedure which generally adds to the patient's ambient level of stress. Since stress and emotional problems often are contributory causes to dysfunctional uterine bleeding, according to Chinese medical theory, additional stress is ill-advised and counterproductive. All too often, D & Cs must be repeated over and over again because the systemic imbalance has not been corrected.

Ovarian wedge resection and hysterectomy are two even more invasive surgical procedures. Chinese medicine believes that scar tissue caused by surgery often itself causes Stagnant Blood due to impaired circulation of the Qi and Blood. In addition, individual meridians may be effected which may eventually lead to lesions in their associated Organs or distant body parts irrigated by these meridians. In the case of hysterectomy, the *Chong, Ren*, Liver, Kidney, and probably Spleen meridians are adversely effected by such surgery. In the case of a partial hysterectomy in which one or both of the ovaries remain, the rise and fall of Qi and Blood continue their monthly cycles but without the discharge of menstruation. Menstruation serves a regulatory function according to Chinese medicine. It discharges Excess Heat along with the menstrual Blood. This Heat can accumulate to cause Stagnant Blood or Stagnant Heat symptoms. In the case of complete hysterectomy, the Yin is usually damaged as evidenced by the tendency for the vaginal tissue to become dry and eventually inflamed in patients who have undergone this procedure.

In general, Chinese medicine has traditionally taught that the energetic balance of the body is founded upon the body's morphological wholeness. Although the body obviously compensates for missing parts and pieces, such "jerry-rigged" balance in only second best. The Uterus is related in Chinese medicine to the Sea of Blood, the Sea of Meridians, the Kidneys, the Liver, and indirectly to the Heart, spinal column, and the Sea of Marrow. The Lower *Dan Tian* is the foundation of Pre Natal Qi and trauma to this area of the body can have long lasting and wide-ranging repercussions. All too often, allopathic practitioners assume that the uterus is only a useless and troublesome piece of excess baggage in a woman who either has had children and does not want more or in a woman who does not wish to have any. This is a very short-sighted point of view. Unfortunately, in America, hysterectomy is all too often the eventual allopathic treatment for dysfunctional uterine bleeding.

Gynecology (*Fu Ke*) is a specialty within Traditional Chinese Medicine which, when compared with allopathic gynecology, is remarkably effective, has few if any side-effects[3], and achieves its results by treating both the Root (*Ben*) and the Branch (*Biao*). In the case of dysfunctional uterine bleeding, the Root is the systemic metabolic imbalance as described by various traditional Chinese medical patterns of disharmony (*Zheng*). That means that Chinese medicine treats the entire person and usually simultaneously addresses other complaints and symptoms beyond just the uterine bleeding. However, traditional Chinese treatment for dysfunctional uterine bleeding is not *just* constitutional or so-called asymptomatic treatment.[4] It does focus on and addresses the primary presenting complaint, i.e. the Branch, the uterine bleeding itself. As we will discuss below, traditional Chinese medical treatment which does not specifically address the uterine bleeding is ineffective and uninformed.

One of the strong points of Chinese medicine is its complex, logical, and clinically-proven physiological theories which explain why things happen on an energetic level. By and large, Western biological science is a description of physical events. Chinese medicine is a description of energetic events. In Chinese medicine, it is believed that this energetic level is deeper than the physical and the penultimate cause of all physical change. The following is a traditional Chinese energetic description of some of the issues and mechanics of dysfunctional uterine bleeding written by Han Bai-ling.[5] This is not just a collection of folk beliefs but is a serious, sophisticated theory of medicine, albeit on a different level of reality than Western medicine, which has been clinically tested for over a millennium by trained medical professionals.[6]

(Excerpted from *Bai Ling Fu Ke [Bai Ling On Gynecology]* by Han Bai-ling)

Gynecological *Beng Lou* is considered a single disorder.[7] Descending *Lou* is light and trickles continuously. *Beng* is heavy and occurs suddenly. These two can also transform into each other. If *Lou* continues for a long time, then the Middle Qi will collapse, the *Chong* and *Ren* will lose their solidity, and this causes *Beng*. Prolonged *Beng* damages the Qi and Blood and eventually must become *Lou*.

The primary cause of *Beng Lou* is the loss of harmonious physiological function among the Five *Zang* which leads to an Internal loss of balance between the Yin and Yang and the Qi and Blood. (This in turn) creates *Beng Lou*. *Beng Lou* can be divided into seven kinds, namely Yin Deficiency, Yang Deficiency, Qi Deficiency, Blood Deficiency, Qi Stagnation, Blood Coagulation, Hot Blood, and so forth. However, (among these) Yin Deficiency will naturally influence Blood Deficiency, just as Blood Deficiency will naturally influence Yin Deficiency. (Likewise,) Yang Deficiency will naturally influence Qi Deficiency and vice versa. Qi Stagnation will naturally influence Blood Coagulation (in the same way that) Blood Coagulation will also influence Qi Stagnation. Hot Blood can be differentiated into Excess and Deficiency varieties. Deficiency Heat is usually (caused by combined) Yin Deficiency and sparse Blood. (Whereas) Excess Heat is usually due to an Excess of Qi, a surplus of Blood, and (simultaneous) Heat.

Zhang Shou-yi says, "When the Blood knows not its position and flows out of its path, this is usually due to Dragon and Lightening Ministerial Fire dredging and dispersing endlessly.[8] Only ingredients that treat the emotions will enable the Liver and Kidneys to grasp and hold the flooding of Deficiency Yang. (This in turn) settles (the Blood's)) unstable home, strengthens its root, and purifies its spring. Without treating the Blood (as such), the bleeding stops of its own accord."[9]

Zhu Dan-xi says: "*Beng* is due to damage to the *Zang Fu* which results in Qi and Blood Deficiency of the *Chong* and *Ren*. These two (ancestral) vessels are the Sea of Channels and Vessels, the pathways of Qi and Blood. The Qi and Blood are circulated externally through the channels and collaterals and circulates internally to nourish the *Zang Fu*. If (they become) excessively exhausted or damaged, then the Qi of the *Chong* and *Ren* becomes Deficient and is unable to produce Blood. Thus the sudden descension of *Beng* is called Suddenly Descending *Beng*."

According to Dai Yuan-ci: "Excessive Blood loss is called *Beng* and it can be either Clear or Turbid or the flushing out of Stagnant Blood. Continuing unabated, *Beng* creates extreme abdominal pain. Most people suffering from Blood diseases have Blood that wants to exit but cannot. It stops in the abdomen and creates Blood Stagnation. This stagnation (in turn) causes nausea and what coagulation is not from Deficiency Cold? For Stagnation causing abdominal pain,

124

moving the Blood stops the pain. When *Beng* creates abdominal pain, holding the Blood will stop the pain."

Shen Zhai says: "Blood hemorrhaging downwards (is due) to the Qi in the internal meridians being ruled by Fire. Of course, Fire (must) also (be differentiated between) Excess and Deficiency."

Every school emphasizes a different pathophysiology for *Beng Lou*. One emphasizes Dragon and Lightening Ministerial Fire or the flooding of Liver/Kidney Deficiency Yang. Another emphasizes damage to the *Zang Fu* with Deficiency of Qi and Blood in the *Chong* and *Ren*. A third emphasizes Deficiency and Excess as the two extremes that can create *Beng* in which abdominal pain due to Deficiency can be stopped by holding the Blood, and abdominal pain due to Stagnant Blood can be stopped by moving the Blood. And yet another emphasizes (the differentiation of) Excess and Deficiency Fire in the causation of *Beng*. The valuable experience collected by our predecessors is excellent material to ponder. When (such theories) are put into practice in the clinic, one can avoid erroneous prescriptions.

Han Bai-ling's above summary of the major classical theories concerning the causation of *Beng Lou* underscores the fact that in different patients dysfunctional uterine bleeding can have a number of different energetic etiologies. Although the primary Chinese diagnostic differentiation of uterine bleeding is between Excess and Deficiency types, successful treatment, whether with herbs or acupuncture, depends upon a more complex and relatively exact diagnosis. In Chinese medicine there is the saying that different diseases may require the same treatment and that the same disease may require different treatments. This means that a single named disease may be caused by any of a number of different patterns of disharmony and a successful treatment must be based on the exact pattern any individual patient is suffering from.

The following case histories have been translated from *Qian Jia Miao Fang (A Thousand Practitioner's Wondrous Prescripsions)*.[10] This is a two volume collection of herbal case histories collected from individual doctors all over China. The case histories presented here exemplify how dysfunctional uterine bleeding is treated with Chinese herbal medicine in China today. In each case, a different Chinese energetic diagnosis has been made, different treatment principles have been deduced, and different herbal prescriptions have been employed. In presenting these case histories we are not suggesting that these are *the* twelve definitive *Zheng* covering dysfunctional uterine bleeding. Rather, they exemplify how twelve different traditional Chinese doctors were able to 1) deduce from the signs and symptoms the precise energetic nature of the imbalance causing the uterine bleeding and 2) write a custom-tailored prescription addressing each issue delineated by the diagnosis.

In several of these cases there is the statement that previous Western and Chinese medical treatment had not achieved satisfactory results. The implication regarding the Chinese treatment is that the previous failures were due to imprecise diagnosis or inexact composition of the prescriptions. When the diagnosis and treatment were correct, the patient responded accordingly. It is hoped that the translation and presentation of these cases may help American practitioners of Traditional Chinese Medicine to more accurately diagnose and treat dysfunctional uterine bleeding. Beyond that, these cases are also examples of the precision and exactitude all American practitioners should strive for in the treatment of all their patients. They are both humbling and encouraging at the same time.

CASE #673

DIAGNOSIS: Hot Blood, Qi Deficiency, & Stagnation blocking the Uterus

TREATMENT PRINCIPLES: Cool the Blood, Benefit the Qi, Enliven the Blood, & Transform Stagnation

PRESCRIPTION: SHEN YU TANG (Curing Saint Decoction) w/ SHI XIAO SAN (Powder for Loss of Smile) w/ modifications

INGREDIENTS: West Radix Codonopsis Pilosulae 30 g., treated Radix Astragali 50 g., cooked Rhizoma Atractylodis Macrocephalae 15 g., Radix Angelicae Sinensis 12 g., Radix Paeoniae Albae 12 g., Cortex Radicis Moutan 10 g., Radix Rehmanniae 30 g., Gelatinum Asini 15 g., (added separately), fresh Pollen Typhae 10 g., (wrapped), cooked Feces Trogopterori 10 g., calcined Concha Ostrea 30 g., (decoct in advance)

Decoct in water and administer this dose daily.[11] For entanglement, add Fructus Seu Semen Amomi 6 g., and Pericarpium Citri Reticulatae 10 g.

Zhang; 30 years old; housecleaner. Initial consultation Feb. 5, 1972

The patient had been widowed for two years and, while still mourning that loss, her son died prematurely. Therefore she was extremely mentally anguished. Gradually her period became irregular and painful. Menstruation arrived early and the flow was heavy as if hemorrhaging. Acute fever caused *Beng* and both Chinese and Western medicine were employed

127

to save her. However, nothing was able to completely stop the flow and a trickle of blood continued. Her face was pale, wan, and dull. Her Spirit was unsettled and the patient was exhausted, dry mouthed, and thirsty. Her menstrual flow was bright red with some purple clots. When her lower abdomen hurt, she did not want to be touched. Her tongue was pale red and the coating was thin and white. Her pulse was wiry, fine and fast. Gynecological examination also revealed cervical dysplasia. Her diagnosis was functional uterine bleeding.[12]

The Powder for Loss of Smile with modifications was given and, after taking two *bao*, purple and black colored blood clots were expelled in significant quantity. Her abdominal pain stopped and the trickle of blood ceased. After two more packets, her *Yuan* Qi revived, her appetite improved, her Spirits clearly improved, and her pulse became supple and harmonious. At this point, Gui Pi Wan and Ren Shen Yang Ying Wan were prescribed for continual improvement.

COMMENT: The Liver is the temperamental organ. Its nature is like a military official. It also stores the Blood. While it is Yin in substance, it is Yang in function. It governs dredging and dispersing as well as insuring the patency of the flow of Qi. The deaths of this patient's husband and son led to Internal Injury by the Seven Emotions, Liver Qi Stagnation, Retarded Qi, and Obstructed Blood. The Liver governs the *Chong* and *Ren* and influences menstruation and its regularity. Chronic Stagnant Liver Qi transforms into Heat which then chases the Blood out of its path and eventually creates "boiling". After heavy blood loss, Blood Deficiency leads to Qi Deficiency. Deficient Qi then has no power to hold the Blood and as a result even more Blood trickles out. With these mutual causes and effects a vicious cycle is created that prolongs bleeding and ultimately results in Deficiency and frailness. Symptoms were bright red menstrual blood accompanied by purple clots and abdominal pain which was sensitive to touch. This indicates Hot Stagnation in the Interior standing and coagulating in the Blood Chamber. Because of heavy Blood loss, the Yin was damaged and thus her face was pale, wan and lacked luster. The patient had little energy, was thirsty, and her pulse was fast (all of which corroborate the damaged Yin).

The herbs that were employed were raw Rehmannia and Moutan to cool the Blood and clear Heat. Dang Gui and Peony nourish the Blood and level the Liver. Codonopsis, Astragalus, and Atractylodes tonify the Spleen and benefit the Qi. Donkey Skin Gel tonifies the Yin and stops bleeding. Pollen Typhae and Feces Trogopterori activate the Blood and disperse Coagulation. Cooked Concha Ostreae consolidates and astringes the Blood to stop bleeding. (Therefore,) this prescription contains the three methods of checking the flow, clearing the spring, and cutting the root. As a result, after (administering the) medication, the Heat in the Blood was leveled and this allowed the bleeding to stop. Dissolving Stagnation allowed new Blood to be created. Solidification of the *Yuan* Qi allowed the Yin and Blood to recover. Not only did the bleeding stop, but the menstruation steadily returned to normal and the patient's overall health returned to her previous norm. In conclusion, this formula is recommended for clinical use whenever one encounters Hot Blood with Qi Deficiency leading to early, heavy, and prolonged menstruation, in which case it gets good results.

CASE #674

DIAGNOSIS: Qi Not Restraining the Blood, *Chong Mai* Not Holding and the Sea of Blood Not Consolidated (Therefore) leading to *Beng*

TREATMENT PRINCIPLES: Benefit the Qi and hold the Blood

PRESCRIPTION: Sheng Qi A Jiao Tang (Decoction of Ginseng, Astragalus, and Donkey Skin Gel)

INGREDIENTS: Red Ginseng tails 9 g., Radix Angelicae Sinensis 9 g., Os Sepiae 9 g., Spirit of Poria 9 g., Gelatinum Asini 9 g., carbonized Radix Sanguisorbae 15 g., Radix Astragali 15 g., Radix Praeparatus Glycyrrhizae 6 g., carbonized Folium Artemesiae Argyi 3 g.

Decoct in water and administer this dose daily. If *Beng* is difficult to stop, (add) Herba Agrimoniae 15 g. and Radix Pseudoginseng 3 g. If the limbs are cold and pulse is slow, (add) Radix Aconiti Carmichaeli 6 g. If there is thirst and the pulse is fast, (add) Radix Scutellariae and Radix Rehmanniae 9 g. @.

Xiang; 36 years old; worker. Admitted to hospital May 24, 1966

The patient's history included nine pregnancies and several miscarriages, including one miscarriage during the winter of the previous year. She had just finished the first trimester of another pregnancy that had resulted in miscarriage and this led to bleeding that had persisted for twenty days despite treatment. At 8 AM on the day she was admitted, hemorrhaging became severe. She was experiencing vertigo, tinnitus, heart palpitations, and had broken out in a cold sweat. Her facial color was pale and wan. Her tongue was pale (with a) white coating and her pulse was minute with a tendency to hesitation. The (TCM) diagnosis was systemic Decline of the *Yuan* Qi and Lack of Consolidation in the *Chong* and *Ren*. Immediately we attempted to benefit the Qi and prevent Blood loss be using Korean Ginseng (6 g.), baked Concha Ostreae (30 g.), and Donkey Skin Gel (15 g.) decocted in water. After taking one packet, the severe bleeding gradually diminished but some Blood flow continued. The patient was dizzy, saw spots, was exhausted, and had a pale tongue. Her pulse was fine and weak. These signs were due to Qi and Blood Deficiency and the treatment principles chosen were to tonify the Qi and consolidate (its) Holding (ability). The herbs used were the Decoction of Ginseng, Astragalus, and Donkey Skin Gel with the addition of Radix Dipsaci and baked Concha Ostreae (15 g. @). After eight packets (*bao*) the illness was cured.

CASE #675

DIAGNOSIS: *Chong Mai* Not Consolidated

TREATMENT PRINCIPLES: Adjust and harmonize the
Chong Mai, benefit the Qi, and stop bleeding

PRESCRIPTION: Fu Fang Shi Wei San (Composite
Powder of Ten Ingredients in Ashes)

INGREDIENTS: Radix Codonopsis Pilosulae 30 g., Radix
Rehmanniae Conquitae 30 g., fresh Cortex
Eucommiae 9 g., Radix Dipsaci 9 g., Rhizoma
Dessicata Zingiberis 3 g., Gelatinum Cornu
Cervi 21 g., Shi Wei San powder[13] 3 g.

Brew up two times per day and take in two separate doses. Add 1 1/2 grams of (Shi Wei San) powder to each decoction. (In addition,) add a few drops of vinegar.

47 year old female whose first visit was on May 25, 1967

(The patient) had been menstruating continuously for forty-three days. Her flow was heavy, the color was red, and there was some clotting. She had had some mild edema (but) her stools and urine were normal. She also had a history of chromic nephritis and coronary heart disease. At the time of

131

treatment, the edema had already been resolved. The (Western) diagnosis was functional uterine bleeding. Her tongue was pale and its coating was white and greasy. Her pulse was deep, thin, grating, and forceless. This was classified as a Lack of Consolidation of the *Chong* and *Ren* and the treatment was aimed at regulating and harmonizing these two channels, benefitting the Qi, and stopping the bleeding. After three days of treatment, her bleeding had essentially stopped. Both sleep and appetite had improved. Her tongue became normal with only a slight greasiness and her pulse was thin and soft. In order to consolidate the *Chong* and *Ren*, the basic prescription was continued without the dried Ginger and following three more *bao* she recovered completely.

COMMENT: In the example above, the patient was already forty-seven years old and the *Chong* and *Ren* were already declining and her constitution was Deficient and weak. Thus the use of Radix Codonopsis and Radix Rehmanniae Conquitae was emphasized in order to benefit the Qi and consolidate the Kidneys. The addition of Cortex Eucommia served to regulate and tonify the *Chong* and *Ren*. The use of Ten Ashes Powder (Shi Wei San) and dried Ginger stopped the bleeding and checked the flow. (Therefore,) the Root and the Branch were treated simultaneously and excellent results were obtained.

CASE #676

DIAGNOSIS: Liver Congestion turning to Fire damaging the *Chong* and *Ren* chasing the Blood out of its path and creating *Beng Lou*

TREATMENT PRINCIPLES: Clear the Liver and cool the Blood

PRESCRIPTION: Qing Gan Zhi Xue Tang (Decoction for

Clearing the Liver and Stopping Bleeding)

INGREDIENTS: Radix Bupleuri 6 g., Radix Paeoniae Albae 4.5 g., Radix Paeoniae Rubrae 4.5 g., Cortex Radicis Moutan 9 g., Folium Mori 6 g., Rhizoma Cyperi 6 g., Radix Rehmanniae 6 g., Radix Scutellariae 6 g., Ramulus Uncariae Cum Uncis 12 g., Radix Angelicae Sinensis 9 g.

Decoct in water for one day's dosage. Modifications: With Liver Yin Deficiency with a fast, thin, wiry pulse and red tongue with little moisture, delete the Bupleurum and Cyperus and add Ligustrum Lucidum and Eclipta, 12 g. @.

27 year old female laborer whose initial consultation was on Dec. 7, 1972

Six days previous to her visit the patient suddenly began bleeding from her vagina. The blood was copious and fresh red in color. Neither Western nor Chinese medicine reduced the bleeding. She was irritable, angry, and dizzy. She suffered from palpitations, fatigue, a bitter taste in her mouth, and was thirsty. Her tongue was pale red and the coating was thin and yellow. Her pulse was wiry and rapid but lacked strength. The (TCM) diagnosis was Liver Fire Chasing the Blood out of its Path. With excessive bleeding the Qi follows the Blood, and is dispersed. The prinicples were to clear the Liver, cool the Blood, and benefit the Qi. In this case, 15 grams of Astragalus were added to benefit the Qi. After one *bao* her bleeding declined. After three (*bao*) the patient was cured.

CASE #677

DIAGNOSIS: Stagnation of Qi and Blood with Insufficiency of Yin and Yang

TREATMENT PRINCIPLES: Tonify the Yang, benefit the Yin, transform Stagnation, and stop bleeding

PRESCRIPTION: Duan Hong Yin (Drink to Cut Off the Red)

INGREDIENTS: Cornu Cervi Pantotrichi 3 g. (place in a separate bag and cook separately), vinegar treated Rhizoma Rhei 6 g., Folium Nelumbinis 30 g., carbonized Trachycarpus Fortunei 10 g., Gelatinum Asini 10 g., (dissolve separately), Radix Pseudoginseng 3 g.(add separately), and Plumula Nelumbinis 6 g.

Decoct in water. Dosage is for one day. Administer two times per day.

40 year old female worker whose initial consultation was on Mar. 4, 1972

The patient had been bleeding in variable amounts for over two years. This was accompanied sometimes with small clots that varied from light to dark (in color). She experienced lower abdominal pain and distention, but when she bled heavily the distention decreased. She also experienced palpitations, insomnia, and headache. Her appetite was good and her bowels and urine were normal. Her tongue was pale red with purple dots on the tip and sides. The coating was thin and white. Her pulse was deep and choppy and her facial color was pale white. She had been recuperating from her illness for the previous eight months.[14] The above decoction was administered three times and the majority of her symptoms subsided. Her pulse became supple and harmonious. (Therefore,) 3 grams of Succinum powder were added to the original prescription and the patient took three more *Bao*. Upon re-examination both the bleeding and the palpitations had stopped. Occasionally the patient still got headaches. The purple dots on her tongue gradually decreased. Her pulse remained supple and harmonious. She went back to the original prescription with the deletion of Rhizoma Rhei and the addition of 30 grams of Ramulus Mori. All the ingredients were ground into powder and 10 grams of this was taken three times per day with water. She continued this regularly for one month after which she returned to work half days. (At this point) she was (considered) completely cured. Two years later her period was normal and she could work full days.

CASE #678

DIAGNOSIS: Qi Stagnation and Blood Deficiency with Stagnation turning to Heat Damaging the *Chong* and *Ren*

TREATMENT PRINCIPLES: Dredge the Liver and liberate Stagnation, nourish and cool the Blood, and stop bleeding

PRESCRIPTION: *Dan Zhi Xiao Yao San Jia Jian* (Moutan and Gardenia Free and Easy Powder with additions and subtractions)

INGREDIENTS: Radix Bupleuri 9 g., Rhizoma Cyperi 12 g., Radix Paeoniae Albae 12 - 15 g., Radix Angelicae Sinensis 10 -12 g., Rhizoma Atractylodis Macrocephalae 9 - 12 g., Sclerotium Poriae Cocoris 12 - 15 g., Cortex Radicis Moutan 9 g., Fructus Gardeniae 9 g., Os Sepiae 12 - 15 g., Radix Rubiae 9 - 12 g., carbonized Pollen Typhae 9 g., raw Concha Ostreae 30 g., Radix Glycyrrhizae 6 g.

Decoct in water for one day's dosage. If the patient has a

tendency to Yin Blood Deficiency, use only 6 grams of Bupleurum but add 15 - 20 grams of raw Rehmannia and 9 - 12 grams of Donkey Skin Gel. For obviously Stagnant Qi with pain and distention in the lower abdomen and a deep, wiry but strong pulse, add 9 - 12 grams of Caulis Perillae which should be infused (at the end) and not decocted.

CASE I: The patient's period had been dripping for forty days and at times there was a sudden gushing of blood. The blood was dark red with clots and occasionally there was abdominal pain and diarrhea. Sometimes the patient experienced heart palpitations. Neither Chinese nor Western medicine had had any effect. The patient's facial color was pale white but she was in good spirits. Her pulse was deep, wiry, and slightly fast, while her tongue was red with a thin, greasy, slightly yellow coat. Her (Western) diagnosis was functional uterine bleeding. (Her TCM diagnosis was) systemic Qi Stagnation and Blood Deficiency with Stagnation Transforming into Fire Damaging the *Chong* and *Ren*. This created the *Beng Lou*. The treatment principles were to relax the Liver and liberate the Stagnation, to nourish and cool the Blood, and to stop bleeding. Modified Moutan and Gardenia Free and Easy Powder was administered three times. After that the bleeding stopped and her abdominal distention and pain lightened. The only problem which persisted was the palpitations. Therefore, 15 grams of Semen Zizyphi Spinosae were added to the original formula and four more *bao* were administered. Following that all her symptoms were relieved and her menstruation returned to normal.

CASE II: 41 year old doctor; initial consultation Oct. 8, 1979

The patient's menstrual flow had continued without ceasing for one month. The flow was fairly heavy and it was deep red in color. The patient also had lower abdominal distention and a sensation of bearing down along with an uncomfortable feeling

136

in her chest and ribs. Her spirits were fairly good. Her pulse was deep, wiry, and fast, while her tongue was red with a thin, yellow coating. Her (Western) diagnosis was functional uterine bleeding. Modified Moutan and Gardenia Free and Easy Powder was prescribed and the bleeding subsided after three *bao*. At this point carbonized Pollen Typhae was deleted and 12 grams of raw Rehmannia were added. After three more *bao* everything had returned to normal.

CASE #679

DIAGNOSIS: Hot and Stagnant Blood with Spleen and Kidney Deficiency

TREATMENT PRINCIPLES: Clear the Heat, activate the Stagnation, tonify the Spleen, and benefit the Kidneys

PRESCRIPTION: Gong Xue Yin (Drink for Working the Blood)

INGREDIENTS: Fructus Rosae Laevigetae 15 g., treated Radix Polygoni Multiflori 15 g., Pericarpium Litchi 15 g., Herba Agrimoniae 15 g., *Chi Di Li*[15] 15 g.

Decoct in water for one day's dosage. For a Hot Blood configuration, add raw Rehmannia, Tuber Ophiopogonis, Cortex Lycii Radicis, Radix Adenophorae, and Fructus Gardeniae. For Stagnant Blood, add Radix Salviae Miltorrhizae, Radix Astragali, and Rhizoma Atractylodis Macrocephalae. For Kidney Yang Deficiency, add Rhizoma Curculingis, Herba Epimedii, and powdered Ginger. For Kidney Yin Deficiency, add Fructus Ligustri Lucidi, Herba Ecliptae, and treated Rhizoma Polygonati.

137

CASE I: 48 year old female worker, first examined Mar. 2, 1971

The patient had suffered from amenorrhea for five years. Suddenly in the last month, she had experienced uterine bleeding. She went to a hospital for treatment but without result. Presently she was still bleeding. Her facial color was pale white. She was exhausted, lacked strength, and experienced dyspnea. Her speech was sluggish (but) she wasn't resting. She was dizzy and did not want to eat or drink. Her tongue was pale with a thin coating. Her pulse was large and deficient. The patient was given the above prescription in its original form and after two *bao* the bleeding stopped. The other symptoms, however, did not decrease and therefore Codonopsis, Astragalus, and Atractylodes were added and three more *bao* were administered. Her Spirit took a change for the better and her appetite and thirst returned to normal. All of her symptoms were relieved following yet another three *bao*. The patient was monitored for one year (following treatment) with no relapse.

CASE II: 21 year old female worker, first examined May 14, 1974.

The day before, the patient suddenly experienced voluminous uterine bleeding. Its color was deep red. There was no change in her symptoms following (Western) injections combined with oral hemostatics. She was restless and feverish, thirsty, and suffered from fitful sleep, vertigo, and headaches. Her urine was yellow and her feces were dry. Her tongue was red with a dry, yellow coating. Her pulse was slippery and fast. The above prescription was therefore employed with the addition of raw Rehmannia, Scutellaria, and Gardenia. After one *bao* over half of the bleeding had stopped and all her other symptoms lightened. She took four more *bao* and achieved a complete cure.[16] Five months later she was re-examined and

138

her menstrual cycle was normal with no recurrence of symptoms.

CASE #680

DIAGNOSIS: Yin Deficiency, Yang Arrested

TREATMENT PRINCIPLES: Moisten the Kidneys, nourish the Liver, benefit the Yin, and harmonize the Blood

PRESCRIPTION: Qing Hai Tang Jia Jian (Decoction for Clearing the Sea w/ modifications)

INGREDIENTS: Radix Rehmanniae Conquitae 24 g., Radix Dioscoreae 12 g., Fructus Corni 12 g., Cortex Radicis Moutan 9 g., Gelatinum Asini 12 g., Tuber Ophiopogonis 12 g., Radix Glehniae 15 g., Rhizoma Atractylodis Macrocephalae 9 g., Radix Paeoniae Albae 15 g., Herba Dendrobii 12 g., Os Draconis 24 g., Folium Mori 24 g., Fructus Ligustri Lucidi 12 g., Herba Ecliptae 12 g.

Decoct in water for one day's dose.

19 year old female, first contracted her illness in the Spring of 1974

(The patient's problem) began with a lengthening of her menstrual cycle (during which she) bled for seven or eight days. During the next month the bleeding continued for ten days. Finally she was trickling blood incessantly throughout the entire month. After close questioning it was discovered that dizziness was interspersed with headaches in the afternoon, spasming tendons, seeing spots, tinnitus which became loudest

139

at dusk, heart palpitations combined with Deficiency irritability, dyspnea accompanied by chest distress, and lumbar and knee pain with aching tendons. In addition, her feces were small and dry, her sleep was short and dream-filled, and the patient was thirsty and easily angered.

It can be seen that the Deficiency was a result of the bleeding and not the primary cause of the disease's Root, but the Branch. Ministerial Fire Flaring Chasing the Blood from its Path was the Root. If one were to only take into account the Deficiency without treating the Root of the Blood loss, then this is (known as) "Discarding the Root and Grasping the Branch" and the treatment will continue without result. Therefore, modified Decoction for Clearing the Sea was administered with the deletion of Atractylodes and the addition of 30 grams of Nodus Nelumbinis. After five *bao* the Floating Deficiency Fire symptoms had greatly decreased and Blood loss had greatly diminished. After ten *bao* the Blood loss had stopped completely, sleeping and eating were excellent, and the patient could move about freely. At this time Folium Mori, Cortex Radicis Moutan, Nodus Nelumbinis, and Os Draconis were removed and Carapax Testudinis, Carapax Amydae, and Concha Ostreae were added to raise the Yin and restore the Yang for a good post-treatment result.

When the patient's next menstruation arrived, everything started fairly normally. However, the patient's mother mistakenly believed advice form others and, thinking that Blood loss must be tonified by Ginseng, Astragalus, Dang Gui, and Lycium berries stewed with chicken, (served her daughter this). This next period showed a large increase in (Blood) volume. The original prescription was again employed with the exchange of raw Rehmannia for cooked Rehmannia. Although the volume decreased, the period lasted nine days. Before the third period we were not concerned about Deficiency and the need to tonify and (herbally) only paid attention to clearing and settling the *Zang Fu*. However, through dietary modification, (we attempted) to moisten and create *Ying* and Blood. In the next premenstrual phase, several *bao* of modified Decoction for Clearing the Sea were given and the period shortened to seven days. (Again) before the following period the same treatment was continued and the bleeding (only) lasted five days. At this time the patient's face appeared very rosy, her vitality had been almost completely restored, and she was already able to resume work. Inquiries over the past six years have revealed continued good health.

EXPLANATION: Modified Decoction for Clearing the Sea is derived from Fu Qing-zhu's Clearing the Sea Pill (Qing Hai Wan). It has been used clinically for nearly forty years and has a truly good effect when treating functional uterine bleeding.

CASE #681

DIAGNOSIS: Qi Deficiency resulting in (the Qi's Inability to Hold the Blood and therefore ceaseless hemorrhage

TREATMENT PRINCIPLES: Benefit the Qi, restrain the Blood, assist Astringing and Consolidation, and stop bleeding

PRESCRIPTION: Gong Xue Tang (Decoction for Working the Blood)

INGREDIENTS: Radix Rehmanniae 20 g., Radix Paeoniae Albae 15 g., Fructus Ligustri Lucidi 15 g., Herba Ecliptae 15 g., fried Flos Sophorae Japonicae 15 g., carbonized Herba Cirsii Japonici 9 g., carbonized Herba Cephalanoplos Segretti 9 g., Carbonized Radix Rubiae 9 g., carbonized Radix Sanguisorbae 15 g.

141

Decoct in water for one day's dosage.

15 year old student.

In March of 1980, due to excessive studying during her menstruation, the patient experienced severe hemorrhaging followed by light bleeding which lasted for over forty days. She was diagnosed and hospitalized for functional uterine bleeding. After receiving Chinese and Western treatment for one month, she checked out of the hospital with her symptoms completely cured. Four days later, (however,) for no apparent reason, she suddenly started bleeding again continuously from her vagina and returned to the hospital. The patient bled continuously, sometimes heavily and sometimes lightly. The blood was pale red, clear, and watery. This was accompanied by dizziness, palpitations, dyspnea, poor sleep, poor appetite, (general) malaise, a sore lumbar region, spontaneous sweating, but no pain in her abdomen. Her pulse was thin and weak and her tongue was pale red with a thin, white coating.

After combining her (various) signs and symptoms, a diagnosis was made of systemic Qi Deficiency Not Holding the Blood to explain the patient's continuous bleeding. The treatment principles were to benefit the Qi and hold the Blood and ingredients were added (to her prescription) to astringe and consolidate and stop bleeding. The prescription was Decoction for Working the Blood. Over twenty *bao* were administered and the illness was completely cured. Inquiries during the following few months showed no sign of relapse.

EXPLANATION: Decoction for Working the Blood is suited for Hot Blood, Qi Deficiency, and Kidney Deficiency patterns of functional uterine bleeding. No matter whether the patient is pubescent, adolescent, middle-aged, or menopausal, with additions and subtractions based on (the individual patient's) signs and symptoms, this adaptable formula will achieve ideal

142

results.

CASE #682

DIAGNOSIS: Deficiency Injury of the Liver and Kidneys, *Chong* and *Ren* Unconsolidated

TREATMENT PRINCIPLES: Tonify the Kidneys, nourish the Blood, consolidate the *Chong*, and regulate the menses

PRESCRIPTION: Bu Shen Gu Jing Tang (Decoction for Tonifying the Kidneys and Consolidating the Menses

INGREDIENTS: Semen Cuscutae 15 g., Radix Dipsaci 12 g., Radix Rehmanniae 9 g., Radix Rehmanniae Conquitae 9 g., Radix Angelicae Sinensis 12 g., Radix Paeoniae Albae 9 g., charred Pollen Typhae 9-12 g., Herba Leonuri 15 g., Cacumen Biotae 12 g., charred Herba Artemisiae Argyi 9 g., Radix Ligusticum Wallachi 6 g., Rhizoma Guanzhong 12-18 g.,

Decoct in water for one day's dose. For Qi Deficiency, add Codonopsis and Astragalus. For Deficiency edema of the face and extremities and abdominal distention, add Poria, Fructus Seu Semen Amomi, and Pericarpium Citri Reticulatae. For incessant hemorrhage with clots, add Radix Pseudoginseng, Donkey Skin Gel, Rhizoma Cyperi, and Feces Trogopterori. For Heat in the Blood portion, add charred Fructus Gardeniae, Herba Agrimoniae, Herba Cirsii Japonici (or Herba Cephalanoplos Segretti).

45 year old patient; initial consultation August 23, 1971

Following a D & C in the latter part of April, the patient bled from the vagina for over a month. An examination of the uterus at that time revealed no obvious changes and the bleeding was successfully treated with a combination of parturition-inducing medicine and Chinese herbs. Later the patient's menstrual cycle shortened with menstruation occurring twice per month. The flow was heavy followed by 10 days or more days of continuous light bleeding. Twice there were no more than a few days between periods. On August 21st, an examination of the endometrium was done and endometrial hyperplasia was confirmed. The (Western) diagnosis was functional uterine bleeding.

The patient suffered from dizziness, fatigue, a sore and aching back, and copious white leukorrhea. Her pulse was thready with the left side being deep, weak, and forceless. Her tongue was pale and purple with a white coat. Her facial color was slightly yellow accompanied by slight edema. These symptoms (when taken together) indicate Deficiency Injury of the Liver and Kidneys and, due to damage from the (previous) pelvic operation (D & C), *Chong* and *Ren* Lacking Solidity accompanied by both Stagnant Blood and Blood Not Returning to the Channels. Treatment was primarily directed at tonifying and benefitting the Liver and Kidneys, consolidating the *Chong,* and regulating the menses. (However,) transformation of Stagnation and strengthening the Spleen (were included to) assist this (process). The prescription chosen was the Decoction for Tonifying the Kidneys and Consolidating the Menses with the addition of 12 grams of Ramus Loranthi Seu Visci, 9 grams of Rhizoma Atractylodis Macrocephalae, 12 grams of Sclerotium Poriae Cocoris, 3 grams of Radix Pseudoginseng, 12 grams of Radix Salviae Miltorrhizae, and 9 grams of Feces Trogopterori. Sixty-two *bao* of the above formula were administered at which time the period returned to normal and all (the patient's) symptoms were relieved. During a follow-up examination in March of 1973, the patient

144

reported that there had been no relapse and that she had been able to continue strenuous work.

CASE #683

DIAGNOSIS: Qi Depletion due to Blood Loss and Insufficient Consolidation and Absorption

TREATMENT PRINCIPLES: Tonify the Qi and consolidate the Blood loss, nourish and absorb the Blood

PRESCRIPTION: Dou Sheng Tang (Decoction of Solitary Root) w/ Tang Kuei Bu Xie Tang Jia Wei (Decoction of Tang Kuei for Tonifying the Blood w/ modifications)

INGREDIENTS: Koren Ginseng 6 g., (decocot separately), honey-baked Radix Astragali 20 g., Radix Angelicae Sinensis 12 g., fried Radix Paeoniae Albae 10 g., charred Human Hair 6 g., roasted Rhizoma Zingiberis 6 g., carbonized Radix Sanguisorbae 12 g., Radix Praeparatus Clycyrrhizae 6 g., Cornu Cervi Pantatrichi 10 g., Gelatinum Asini 12 g., (melt separately)

Decoct in water for one day's dosage.

45 year old, married female; initial consultation May 25, 1967

Following her menses, the patient experienced sudden and continuous vaginal bleeding. The blood was large in volume, pale in color, and without clots. She experienced dizziness, dyspnea, languid speech, fatigue, (spontaneous) perspiration, and trembling. She also had palpitations and agitation as well as lack of both appetite and thirst even though her lips and mouth were dry. Upon examination, her pulse was found to be

145

hollow and her tongue pale with a thin, white coating. Her facial color was white and without luster and she lacked Spirit. Her voice was low and had a groaning quality to it and her extremities lacked warmth. Thus, her Qi had become depleted due to Blood loss and consolidation and assimilation were insufficient. Therefore *Beng* resulted. Treatment was directed at tonifying the Qi and consolidating the Blood as well as the nourishing and absorbing of the Blood. The Decoction of Solitary Root in conjunction with the Decoction of Dang Gui for Tonification of the Blood and added flavors were employed.

After four *bao* (of the above), the patient returned to the hospital by foot. Her bleeding had ceased and she had a healthy complexion. Her Spirit was comparatively strong and all of her symptoms were entirely gone. Upon palpation, however, her pulse was (still found to be) rather fine and weak. (In addition,) her tongue was pale red with a thin, white coating. It was (therefore) determined that she was (still) weak following her illness and she was urged to improve her nutrition, rest, and to temporarily avoid sex. Medication was suspended and observation was discontinued. In a follow-up call in August of 1967, the patient reported no (further) recurrence of her symptoms and that her menses were normal and her constitution strong.

COMMENT: This (case) is an example of the Chinese medical pattern of *Xue Beng* or Avalanche Bleeding where, following the menses, there is sudden, incessant bleeding. The Qi (thus becomes) depleted due to Blood loss and there is hemorrhaging with the intensity of waves in a river. The Decoction of Solitary Root, (when) employed immediately, checks Blood loss and quells Rebellion, while the Decoction of Tang Kuei for Tonification of the Blood tonifies the Qi, generates Blood, and assists in consolidating Blood loss. The concept is that since Blood has form, it cannot be quickly generated, but since Qi is formless, it can and should be immediately (generated) to consolidate (the loss). The addition of roasted Ginger and baked Licorice warms the Middle and holds the Blood. Donkey Skin Gel and Peony nourish the Yin and tonify the Blood. Carbonized Radix Sanguisorbae and carbonized Human Hair rescue the Blood and stop bleeding. Deer Antler tonifies and Yang and nourishes the Kidneys and assists in the generation of Blood. The principles are to create Yang, generate Yin, and regulate and restain the *Chong* and *Ren* which (will therefore) stop the bleeding. Thus, these ingredients, when used in conjunction, serve to return the Qi and create the Blood (thereby) consolidating and restraining the *Chong* and *Ren*. Therefore *Xue Beng* subsides on its own.

CASE #684

DIAGNOSIS: Flaring Liver causing Hot Blood

TREATMENT PRINCIPLES: Cool the Blood and clear the Liver

PRESCRIPTION: Qing Hai Tang (Decoction for Clearing the Sea)

INGREDIENTS: Fried Radix Paeoniae Albae 30 g., carbonized Flos Sophorae 18 g., Folium Mori 15 g., Herba Leonuri 15 g., carbonized Radix Scrophulariae 15 g., carbonized Receptaculum Nelumbinus 30 g., carbonized Cortex Radicis Moutan 18 g., Caulis Bambusae In Taeniam 9 g., sweet Flos Chrysanthemi 5 g.

Decoct in water and administer as one day's dose. If there is severe bleeding the day before menstruation, add Rhizoma Coptidis, etc. to cool the Blood and clear the Liver to prevent (the Blood) from boiling over. If (severe bleeding) follows the menses, add Fructus Lycii, Rhizoma Polygonati, Flos and Cortex Albizziae, Tuber Ophiopogonis, and Donkey Skin Gel to nourish the Yin and revive and consolidate the Liver.

49 year old, female office workier; initial consultation July 5, 1978

The patient complained of a history of uterine bleeding. She had received a D & C and been diagnosed as having functional uterine bleeding. For some time her condition had been stable. However, in the last year her old symptoms had returned. Her menstrual flow was extremely heavy and she had experienced incessant spotting for two or three months. Her complexion was flushed red. She was easily irritated and suffered from insomnia. Her tongue was red with a thin coating, while her pulse was fine, thin, *Dai*[17], and fast. During menopause, women at the age of forty-nine experience *Tian Kui* [18] and the exhaustion of both Kidney and Liver Yin. While, in addition, in the heat of summer, Summer Heat Evil may contribute to the boiling of the Sea of Blood. The menstrual flow will be heavy and the color bright (red). Thus the immediate principles are to clear the Source, check the flow, and calm the Sea of Blood and it is appropriate to use Qing Hai Wan (Clearing the Sea Pills) as a basis to yield the Decoction for Clearing the Sea, to be administered in five doses.

The patient's second visit was on July 27th. The source had been cleared and the flow checked, and, with the administration of large doses (of herbs,) the Sea of Blood was calmed. The blood volume had lessened. However, it was essential to coninue clearing the *Lou* through the next cycle. The primary treatment principles at that time were to continue ensuring that the Uterus was fully closed and cooled and to ensure consolidation of the Sea of Blood. 12 grams of Fructus Lycii , 9 grams of Rhizoma Anemarrhenae, and 9 grams of

Cortex Radicis Lycii were added to the above prescription and another four *bao* were administered. On October 23rd, the patient reported that through the succeeding four cycles the bleeding had changed and that during (the month of October) there had been a striking decrease in the Blood volume. The duration of the menses was also shorter and her menstruation had been essentially normal. Following her flow, however, the Blood had left and the Blood had been injured, her Heart and Liver Channels were both exhausted, and she experienced palpitation, dream-disturbed sleep, and restlessness. Thus it became necessary to nourish the Heart and to rescue and aid the Liver in consolidating its defense. The formula employed consisted of 9 grams of raw Radix Paeoniae Albae, Radix Astragali, Tuber Ophipogonis, Fructus Lycii, Sclerotium Poriae Cocoris, and Radix Codonopsis, 15 grams of Fructus Zizyphi Sattivae, 12 grams of Herba Leonuri, 6 grams of Radix Glycyrrhizae, and 30 grams of Fructus Tritici Levis. The patient took four *bao* and was fine thereafter.

CASE #685

DIAGNOSIS: Hot Blood in the *Chong* and *Ren*

TREATMENT PRINCIPLES: Clear Heat and cool the Blood

PRESCRIPTION: Jia Wei Bai Dai Tang (Decoction of Pulsatilla and Sanguisorbae with added flavors)

INGREDIENTS: Radix Pulsatillae 90 g., Radix Sanguisorbae 60 g., carbonized Radix Rehmanniae 30 g., White sugar 60 g.

Decoct the first three ingredient first. Then add the White Sugar. Begin administering the prescription on the first day of the period and daily thereafter. Continue for several *bao* after

149

the bleeding ceases to consolidate the treatment.

18 year old, unmarried female, first examined in March of 1974

The patient complained of incessant vaginal bleeding for over twenty days. The color of the Blood was red and its volume was heavy. The patient's face and lips were a sallow white. Her limbs lacked strength and for three months she had been unable to do manual labor. Gynecological examination (resulted in a Western) diagnosis of adolescent functional uterine bleeding. The patient was prescribed Gui Pi Tang (Decoction for Restoring the Spleen) in combination with Si Wu Tang (Decoction of Four Ingredients) with the addition of Herba Artemesiae Argyi. More than fifty *bao* (of this) were administered. In addition, the patient received progesterone along with (the above) hemostatic herbs but the results were unsatisfactory. (Therefore,) the Decoction of Pulsatilla and Sanguisorba with added flavors was administered. After one *bao*, a reduction in bleeding was evident and following the second *bao* the bleeding stopped. While after five *bao*, the patient had recovered completely. On a subsequent visit, she reported that her periods were regular and that her constitution was strong.

The Decoction of Pulsatilla and Sanguisorba with modifications gets good results in the treatment of both pubescent and (adult) functional uterine bleeding. Its ingredients are: Radix Pulsatillae, which has a Bitter, Cold nature and vitalizes Stagnant Blood, clears Heat, and cools the Blood as well as having antibiotic and anti-inflammatory properties; Radix Sanguisorbae, which has a Bitter taste and slightly Cold nature, is sinking and descends into the Lower Burner, is primarily used to clear Heat and cool the Blood, whose fried and carbonized form has hemostatic effects, and which is an important herb in the treatment of *Beng Lou*; White Sugar, which is Sweet, slightly Warm, regulates and harmonizes the Spleen and Stomach, and moves the Blood and transforms Stagnation. The use of these three ingredients together ensure success.

CASE #686

DIAGNOSIS: *Chong* and *Ren* Deficient and Cold with Stasis and Obstruction of the Uterus

TREATMENT PRINCIPLES: Warm the Channels, disperse Cold, nourish the Blood, rid Obstruction

PRESCRIPTION: Wen Jing Tang (Decoction for Warming the Channels)

INGREDIENTS: Fructus Evodiae 6 g., Radix Angelicae Sinensis 12 g., wine-cooked Radix Paeoniae Albae 12 g., large Radix Ligustici Wallichi 5 g., Radix Codonopsis (from Lu-an, Shanxi region) 12 g., Szechuan Ramulus Cinnamomi 5 g., Gelatinum Asini 15 g. (dissolved separately), powdered Cortex Radicis Moutan 10 g., Rhizoma Recens Zingiberis 3 slices, Radix Praeparatus Glycyrrhizae 5 g.

Decoct in water for one day's dose.

24 year old female worker; first examined Oct. 5, 1973

The patient had been taking birth control medication since her marriage almost one year ago. As a result of stopping the medication, she experienced sudden vaginal bleeding which continued unabated. This condition persisted for three months up through the time of the examination. The color of the Blood was dark. Its quantity was small and there were clots

151

and lower abdominal pain and coldness. The patient was exhausted. Her lumbar legion and knees were also mildly sore. In the gynecological department of a hospital she had been diagnosed as suffering from functional uterine bleeding, though repeated administration of estrogen, androgen, and progesterone yielded no cure. (Therefore,) she came for (TCM) treatment.

The patient's pulse was fine and wiry and her tongue was pale with a thin, white coating. Her facial color was a lusterless, sallow yellow. (These) were caused by Deficiency Cold of the *Chong* and *Ren* thus obstructing the Uterus and resulting in the incessant trickling of Blood from the vagina. Treatment was directed at warming the Channels, dispersing Cold, nourishing the Blood, and ridding Obstruction. Thus the Decoction for Warming the Channels was prescribed and following ten *bao* the bleeding stopped and the illness was cured.

A follow-up examination in May of 1978 revealed no recurrence of the previous symptoms. In January of 1974, the patient ceased menstruating due to pregnancy and in October of the same year delivered a baby boy. Both the mother and child were healthy.

COMMENT: This is an example of the *Beng Lou* pattern of Traditional Chinese Medicine. The symptoms may vary in terms of severity and as to whether they are chronic or acute and each possibility (requires) distinct treatment principles. When the pulse and symptoms of this example were considered together and an etiology carefully ascertained, it was (diagnosed according to TCM) as Deficient and Cold *Chong* and *Ren* with Stagnation in the Uterus. The prescription was based on the time-honored use of Zhang Zhong-jing's Decoction for Warming the Channels from the *Jin Gui Yao Lue*. In (this prescription,) Evodia and Cinnamon warm the Channels and disperse Cold. Dang Gui, Peony, and Donkey

Skin Gel moisten the Yin and tonify Blood. Ligusticum and Moutan assist Cinnamon in moving the Blood and ridding obstruction. Codonopsis and treated Licorice along with fresh Ginger tonify the Qi and harmonize the Middle as well as regulate the source of Blood generation. In combination, this is an important prescription for warming the Channels, nourishing the Blood, ridding Stagnation, and generating new Blood. Thus its clinical application is wide-ranging.

Readers familiar with the Chinese herbal formulae popularized in the books and periodicals published by the Oriental Healing Arts Institute (OHAI) will notice that the dosages of individual formulae given above are much larger than those given in OHAI materials. Also there is a much greater use of styptic or hemostatic herbs. The formulae given above are from contemporary Chinese TCM[19] practitioners and reflect the accepted current norm for TCM herbalism. Traditional Chinese Medicine is a Rational style of medicine.[20] Its treatment are derived from principles in turn deduced from the energetic diagnosis. TCM diagnosis is based on the discrimination of named patterns of disharmony or *Bian Zheng*. The so-called "ancient formulae" (*Gu Fang*) promulgated by OHAI are based on an Empirical style of Chinese medicine popular in Japan and to some extent in Taiwan, which, it should be remembered, was under Japanese control for most of the first half of this century. Diagnosis in this style, known in Japanese as *Kanpo Yaku*, is not based on named patterns but on the patient's conformation. If the patient looks like this and this and these signs and symptoms and especially this or that abdominal conformation, use this or that formula. In other words, instead of diagnosing a patient as suffering from Liver Qi Congestion with Spleen Deficiency, patients of this style would be diagnosed as Minor Bupleurum (Decoction) conformation. In general, it is my observation that this approach places its primary emphasis on rebalancing the constitution Root as opposed to alleviating conditional

153

symptoms.

In the TCM case histories given above, there is in each case a statement of therapeutic principles believed necessary to correct the imbalance identified and stated in the diagnosis. In case #678, the diagnosis was Stagnation of Qi and Blood and Insufficiency of Yin and Yang. The principles given to redress this disorder were, therefore, to tonify Yang, benefit the Yin, transform Stagnation, *and* stop bleeding. Based on these four principles, ingredients were chosen to accomplish each of these goals. Of the seven ingredients, four of them are categorized as hemostatics: Folium Nelumbinus, carbonized Trachycarpus, Donkey Skin Gel, and Radix Pseudoginseng. The inclusion of hemostatic ingredients is, in my experience, the difference between successful and unsuccessful treatment. In case #679, the well-known formula for Qi Stagnation and Blood Deficiency with Congestion transforming into Heat, Dan Zhi Xiao Yao San, is the prescription selected as the foundation of the treatment. Yeung Him-che, in *Handbook of Chinese Herb Formulas,* Vol II, lists as one of the indications of this formula uterine bleeding.[21] However, in my experience, this formula without the addition of hemostatic herbs does not get good results in such cases. The modified version of this fomula used in case #679 includes three ingredients not found in the unmodified version: Os Sepiae, carbonized Pollen Typhae, and raw Concha Ostreae. It is the addition of these herbs that, in my opinion, made this formula specifically appropriate for treating the uterine bleeding described in this case.

Chinese is a very difficult language to translate into English. The basic structure of the two languages is totally dissimilar. English is linear and denotative. Chinese is eliptical and connotative. English is based on a mechanistic theory of causation and Chinese is based on codependent arising. Some Western practitioners, in attempting to read Chinese treatment principles, may interpret the principles in case #679 as dredge the Liver, liberate Stagnation, nourish the Blood, and cool the Blood *to* stop bleeding. However, as the formula itself clearly demonstrates, the principles should be read as dredge the Liver, liberate Stagnation, nourish the Blood, cool the Blood, *and* stop bleeding. In the treatment of hemorrhagic disorders, the stopping of bleeding is always a first priority since the Blood is a Pure Substance. American practitioners are sometimes not clear about the conceptual differences between *Kanpo Yaku* and TCM herbalism and the treatment of hemorrhagic disorders is an important area where such differences should be clearly distinguished. It is my experience that the TCM approach is clinically superior for treating *Biao* or Branch symptoms. However, the TCM approach requires the use of individually dispensed, bulk herbal ingredients. Dessicated powdered formulae do not allow for the customized modification which is the forte of the TCM approach. In chronic cases where the treatment of the *Ben* or Root is sufficient, dessicated powdered formulae may be adequate or even preferable, but in cases where the *Biao* is equally as important as the *Ben*, I recommend the use of bulk herbs.

Dysfunctional uterine bleeding is also amenable to treatment by acupuncture and moxibustion. Since acupuncture theory emphasizes the flow of Qi and Blood within the Channels and Collaterals, the diagnosis of *Beng Lou* in acupuncture stresses Injury to the *Chong* and *Ren* which therefore fail to control the Blood.[22] Drs. Lian Qiu-mao and Ming Su-xin of the Nanjing College of Traditional Chinese Medicine divide *Beng Lou* into Excess and Deficiency types and then subdivide these into seven separate *Zheng*. The three Deficiency types of *Beng Lou* according to Lian and Ming are: 1) Spleen Qi Deficiency rendering the Spleen Incapable of holding the Blood within its Path; 2) Kidney Yang Deficiency weakening the Kidney's Consolidating and Grasping Function resulting in Dysfunction of the *Chong* and *Ren*; and 3) Kidney Yin Deficiency with Deficiency Fire effecting the *Jing* and Blood

155

forcing them out of their Paths. The four Excess types they give are 1) Hyperactivity of Yang or pathogenic Heat injuring the *Chong* and *Ren* causing Hot Blood to move recklessly; 2) Stagnation of Liver Qi Transforming into Fire leading to the Dysfunction of the Liver in storing Blood; 3) Accumulation of Damp Heat in the Lower *Jiao* injuring the *Bao Mai*[23] thus causing uterine bleeding; and 4) Internal Stagnation of the Blood causing the Blood to flow outside its proper course.[24]

These seven *Zheng* are all standard TCM patterns of disharmony and their differential diagnosis can be found in a number of English language sources. [25] However, a description of the specific types of bleeding one would expect with each of these etiologies is germane. In Spleen Qi Deficiency, the bleeding is profuse or lingering and its color is light red. In Kidney Yang Deficiency, the bleeding is basically the same. In Kidney Yin Deficiency *Beng Lou*, the bleeding is scanty or lingering and the blood is bright red in color. Among the Excess varieties, in Hot Blood *Beng Lou*, one can expect profuse bleeding, deep red in color, of thick consistency, possibly accompanied by a fetid smell. In Accumulation of Internal Heat, Lian and Ming do not specifically describe the discharge. However, in discussing the preceding *Zheng* they say that thick, fetid blood is characteristic of Heat. In Damp Heat bleeding, the blood is profuse or continuous and lingering. It is also dark red but is not thick. And in Stagnant Blood *Beng Lou*, the blood contains clots.[26]

As for acupuncture treatment protocols, for all four Excess varieties, Lian and Ming suggest using *Qi Hai* (CV 6), *San Yin Jiao* (Sp 6), and *Yin Bai* (Sp 1) as the foundation to which other points may be added depending upon the specific *Bian Zheng*. For Hot Blood *Beng Lou*, add *Xue Hai* (Sp 10) and *Shui Quan* (Ki 5). All points should be needled with *Xie Fa* (reducing technique) and no moxa should be applied. For Internal Heat, add *Tai Chong* (Liv 3), *Zhi Gou* (TH 6), and *Da*

156

Dun (Liv 1) with *Xie Fa* and no moxa. For Damp Heat bleeding, add *Zhong Ji* (CV 3), and *Yin Ling Quan* (Sp 9) with *Xie Fa* and no moxa. Add for Stagnant Blood *Beng Lou*, add *Di Ji* (Sp 8) *Qi Chong* (St 30), and *Chong Men* (Sp 12), again with *Xie Fa* and no moxa. In addition, if Heat is severe, add *Da Zhui* (GV 14) and *Qu Chi* (LI 11) and treat up to three times per day. For irritability, add *Jian Shi* (Per 5). For excessive leukorrhea accompanying Damp Heat *Beng Lou*, add *Ci Liao* (Bl 32). For costal and hypochondral distention due to Liver Fire, add *Shan Zhong* (CV 17), *Qi Men* (Liv 14), and *Yang Ling Quan* (GB 34). And finally, for abdominal pain with pressure due to Stagnant Blood, add *He Gu* (LI 4), *Zhong Ji*, and *Si Man* (Ki 14).

For the three Deficiency patterns, Lian and Ming suggest a basic protocol consisting of *Guan Yuan* (CV 4), *San Yin Jiao*, *Shen Shu* (Bl 23), and *Jiao Xin* (Ki 8). For Spleen Qi Deficiency, add one or more of the following as appropriate: *Qi Hai, Pi Shu* (Bl 20), *Ge Shu* (Bl 17), and *Zu San Li* (St 36). Needle with *Bu Fa* (tonification technique) and/or moxa. For Kidney Yang Deficiency, add *Qi Hai, Ming Men* (GV 4) and *Fu Liu* (Ki 7) with *Bu Fa* and definitely moxa at least *Ming Men, Shen Shu*, and *Guan Yuan*. For Kidney Yin Deficiency *Beng Lou*, and *Ran Gu* (Ki 2) and *Yin Gu* (Ki 10). Reduce *Ran Gu* and tonify *Yin Gu*. If diarrhea accompanies either Spleen Qi or Kidney Yang Deficiency, add *Tian Shu* (St 25). For insomnia due to Yin Deficiency, add *Shen Men* (Ht 7) and *An Mian* (Extra). For night sweats due to Yin Deficiency, add *Yin Xi* (Ht 6). And for sore and weak low back and knees due to Kidney Deficiency, add *Yao Yan* (Extra) for the back and *Xi Yan* (Extra) for the knees.

As with the herbal prescriptions given above, these acupuncture protocols are based on the rather precise differentiation of the various patterns of disharmony responsible for *Beng Lou*. These protocols are more exact and

157

sophisticated than those found in *Essentials*[27], *Comprehensive*[28], *A Barefoot Doctor's Manual*[29], or other such acupuncture treatment formularies available in English. For several years, my acupuncture treatments for uterine bleeding have been only moderately effective. Using simpler protocols than above, some patients would get better quickly and some would not. Using these more precise protocols, my success rate in treating uterine bleeding with acupuncture has considerably improved. My one addition to the above points is the mention of *Bai Hui* (GV 20) with moxa in cases of recalcitrant uterine bleeding due to Spleen Qi or Kidney Yang Deficiency. Also I have found that when using *Yin Bai*, a better effect is gotten with *direct* moxibustion in Excess scenarios of *Beng Lou*. My belief is that this point strongly catalyzes the Spleen's ability to hold the Blood and that, since the Heat is not in the Spleen, it is acceptable and even preferable to moxa this point while reducing with needles the other points. In my experience, needling this point or treating it with indirect moibustion does not get the immediate and pronounced results direct moxibustion does.

It is my conclusion that herbs and acupuncture in tandem work best for the three Excess varieties of *Beng Lou*. Since the bleeding is profuse and since it may be accompanied by pain, aggressive therapy to treat the Branch is called for. As Dr.s Lian and Ming point out: "Emergency measures must be adopted, e.g. in a case of massive haemorrhage such as uterine or stomach, the bleeding (*Biao*) must be stopped, no matter what the *ben*."[30] In Spleen Deficiency and Kidney Deficiency I rely more heavily on herbal therapy, although I have found that giving patients *Ibuki* moxa to do at home is a useful adjunct for increasing effectiveness and for involving the patient more fully in her treatment. In addition, in cases of imminent collapse of Yang due to extreme Deficiency due in turn to Blood loss, moxibustion at *Bai Hui* is also a useful adjunct to herbal therapy. In cases of Yin Deficiency, I have

158

not found acupuncture to be cost or time effective and therefore I do not generally add it to the treatment plan in such cases.

Once the uterine bleeding has been brought under control by professional therapy, more emphasis should be placed on the patient's diet and lifestyle. Spleen Qi Deficiency may be constitutional or it may be caused by improper diet and/or excessive fatigue or stress. No matter what the cause, proper diet and minimization of fatigue and stress are absolutely necessary in order to consolidate the treatment and redress the Root. Proper diet for Spleen Deficiency includes avoiding or minimizing cold, frozen, and raw foods and drinks and sugar and sweets. In Kidney Yang Deficiency, rest is very important, as are avoiding alcohol, coffee, black tea, sugar and sweets, recreational drugs, and sex. In Kidney Yin Deficiency, avoiding the same foods and drinks is suggested. In addition, even greater emphasis should be placed on programmed relaxation, rest, and reduction of stress. The patient should refrain from too much reading, thinking, or entertainment such as movies, TV, or loud, exhilirating music.

In Hot Blood *Beng Lou*, it is important to avoid or minimize the ingestion of Hot, Spicy, pungent foods and greasy, oily foods. In *Prince Wen Hui's Cook*, I have given a case history of a woman who had Hot Blood *Beng Lou* due to overeating chicken.[31] Chicken and some shellfish, such as shrimp, can cause Hot Blood. In Stagnation of Liver Qi transforming into Fire, one should avoid coffee, alcohol, greasy and oily foods, Hot, Pungent foods, and also and most importantly one *must* minimize stress through lifestyle simplification *and* practice programmed relaxation. With Damp Heat in the Lower *Jiao*, one should avoid Hot, Pungent foods, greasy foods, alcohol, sugar, and dairy. The patient should also be advised to get adequate, regular exercise. Stagnant Blood in the Lower Burner in American patients is most ofter due to Liver

159

Congestion, abdominal surgery, abortions, and the treatment of pelvic, vaginal, and urinary tract infections with antibiotics. The same foods which aggravate Liver Qi given above should be avoided and the patient should get regular exercise and relaxation. Ginger compresses applied to the lower abdomen can also be useful in the treatment of Stagnant Blood and to return responsibility to the patient. In all *Zheng* aggravated by stress, full body, relaxation massage is also useful preventively and as an adjunct to remedial treatment.

It is obvious from the above that Chinese medicine addresses the whole person in treating dysfunctional uterine bleeding. As several of the case histories point out, Chinese-style therapy is able to successfully treat some patients in whom Western allopathic medicine has been ineffective. In addition, Chinese medicine does not cause irreversible harm to the patient in the course of treatment. It is my opinion that Chinese medicine, including herbal therapy and acupuncture, should be resorted to first before Western-style allopathy for the treatment of dysfunctional uterine bleeding. If it fails to correct the situation with its conservative therapy, then more heroic measures can be taken.[32]

ENDNOTES

1   Berkow, Robert, Talbott, John, et.al., *The Merck Manual*, (Merck Sharp & Dohme Research Laboratories), Rahway, NJ, 1977. p. 899

2   Long, James, *The Essential Guide to Prescription Drugs*, (Harper & Row), NY, etc., 1985, 333 & 334

3   Properly prescribed Chinese herbal and acupuncture treatment should be without side-effects. If side-effects occur, treatments must be adjusted until they are eliminated. According to Huang Pao-chin, treatment with certain herbs renders the patient incapable of eating certain foods for the rest of their lives. Once treated with these herbs, if the patient were to eat one of these foods, it would create a systemic imbalance. However, also according to Dr. Huang, these herbs are seldom, if ever, used because of this complication.

4   Asymptomatic or Root treatment is becoming more and more popular in Japan. For a discussion of this approach to Oriental medicine see: Felt, Robert, *Redwing Reviews*, Redwing Book Co., Brookline, MA, December, 1985, p. 2 & 3

5   Han Bai-ling, *Bai Ling Fu Ke*, (Heilongjiang People's Press), Haerbin, PRC, 1983, p. 63

6   That some allopathic physicians consider Traditional Chinese Medicine a collection of superstitious folk beliefs is evident from an editorial written by Dr. George Ulett appearing in the *Southern Medical Journal* and quoted in the *American Journal of*

Acupuncture, Felton, CA, Vol 13, #3, Sept., 1985, p. 298

7   These two characters, pronounced *Beng* and *Lou* respectively, describe qualitative different kinds of uterine bleeding as defined in this text. When used in combination, they form a technical term in TCM literature which essentially means uterine bleeding.

8   This is a difficult passage to translate. It is our reading that Dragon and Lightening refer to Excess *Ming Men Huo* which, when manifest in the Liver, causes excessive dredging and dispersing, thus causing Kidney Liver Yin Deficiency. The Yang floats or floods up due to this Deficiency, which in turn unsettles the Spirit residing in the Heart. The Heart governs the Blood and due to this imbalance loses its control.

9   In other words, by using Yin tonics, which indirectly control the Yang, and Spirit-calming herbs, one can control the Blood without using herbs which specifically or directly act on the Blood portion.

10   Li Wen-liang, Qi Qiang, et.al., *Qian Jia Miao Fang*, (Liberation Army Publishing), Beijing, 1985

11   The text is clear in stating that the formula given is a one day's dose. It does not specify, however, how many times per day this dose should be apportioned nor whether it should be taken before or after meals, etc. It is generally believed in Chinese medicine that formulae whose effects must manifest in the lower half of the body should be taken before meals so that the food eaten after pushes the herbs' energy down with peristalsis.

12   Typically, in contemporary TCM hospitals in China, two diagnoses are written down on the patient's chart: 1) a Western medical diagnosis and 2) a TCM diagnosis. The Chinese term here is an exact translation of functional uterine bleeding. Therefore, although we believe that dysfunctional uterine bleeding is the more correct term, we have translated this term as the Chinese have written it.

13   Ingredients in Powder of Ten Ashes:

> Herba Seu Radix Cirsii Japonici
> Folium Nelumbinis
> Rhizoma Imperatae
> Rhizoma Rhei
> Skin of Petiolus Trachycarpus
> Herba Cephalanoploris
> Cacumen Biotae
> Rhizoma Rubiae
> Fructus Gardeniae
> Cortex Radicis Moutan

All ingredients in this formula are to be carbonized.

14   I.e., the patient was on sick leave, one of the few luxuries Chinese can afford with their system of socialism

15   We have been unable to identify this ingredient. Several Chinese apothecaries and *Lao Yi Sheng* or "old doctors" have not been able to shed any light on it. It may, in fact, be a typographical error. Second edition: Fructus Tribuli Terrestris

16   In my opinion, Chinese case histories often tend to be simplistic and over-emphsize the major complaint.

According to Michael Broffman, a patient should not be considered cured for at least one year without relapse or transformation. Even then, American patients, by and large, are looking for more subtle levels of health and well-being than generally the Chinese have the time and resources to address.

17   *Dai Mai*: a regularly intermittent pulse which is rather slow and weak. It is often encountered in cases of Deficient *Zang* Qi and heart disease.

18   "Regarding the problem of *Tian Kui*, doctors throughout the dynasties have stated their individual and differing opinions. Some feel that *Tian Kui* is Kidney Water. Some consider it Yin *Jing*. And others think it is menstruation itself. This author feels that *Tian Kui* results from the combination of Prenatal basic substance from which the body is created and the Postnatal *Jing Qi* which is transformed from Water and Grain and which nourishes the body. Both together serve to insure the development of *Tian Kui*. When females reach approximately the age of 14, all five *zang* are mature. The Kidney Qi is full and *Tian Kui* development is also mature. *Ren Mai* Qi communicates, *Chong Mai* Blood fluorishes, and this creates the menstrual flow and the capacity for child-bearing." Han Bai-ling, op.cit., p. 7

19   TCM, or Traditional Chinese Medicine, is a particular stype of Chinese medicine. It is the state-approved version practiced in the People's Republic of China. This style is based on Confucianism and the materialism of the *Han Xue Pai* movement of the Qing dynasty and on the dialectical materialism of Communism. That Chinese medicine is not a single orthodoxy is ably proven by Paul Unschuld in *Medicine*

in China, A History of Ideas, (UC Press), Berkeley, etc., 1985

20   For a fuller exposition of the dichotomy between Rational and Empirical medicine, see H.L. Coulter's *Divided Legacy: A History of The Schism of Medical Thought*, (Weekawken Book Co.), Washington, D.C., 1975

21   Yeung Him-che, *Handbook of Chinese Herbs and Formulas*, Vol. II, (self-published), LA, 1985, p. 72

22   Lian Qiu-mao & Ming Su-xin, *The Nanjing Seminars, The Journal of Chinese Medicine*, UK, 1984, p. 8

23   "The *bao mai* is a collateral of the uterus. It flows just inside and outside the uterus. There are two collaterals connecting the *bao mai* with the HE (Heart) and KID (Kidneys) respectively." Ibid., p. 26

24   Ibid., p. 8 & 9

25   Porkert, Manfred, *The Essentials of Chinese Diagnosis*, (Chinese Medicine Publishers), Zurich, 1983

        Kaptchuk, Ted, *The Web That Has No Weaver*, (Congden & Weed), NY, 1983

        Cheung, C.S. & Lai, Yat-ki, *Principles of Dialectical Differential Diagnosis and Treatment of Traditional Chinese Medicine*, (Traditional Chinese Medicinal Publishers), SF, 1980

26   Lian & Ming, op.cit., p. 9 & 10

27   Anon. Committee, *Essentials of Chinese Acupuncture*,

(Foreign Language Press), Beijing, 1980

28   Anon. Committee, *Acupuncture, A Comprehensive Text*, trans. & ed. by John O'Connor & Dan Bensky, (Eastland Press), Chicago, 1981

29   Anon. Committee, *A Barefoot Doctor's Manual*, (Cloudburst Press), Seattle, 1977

30   Lian & Ming, op.cit., p. 86

31   Flaws, Bob & Wolfe, Honora Lee, *Prince Wen Hui's Cook*, (Paradigm Publications), Higganum, CT, 1983, p. 30

32   Case history #679 in the *Qian Jia Miao Fang* includes a synopsis of research data compiled on the Chinese treatment of *Beng Lou* in the hospital in which the author of this particular case worked. In 83 cases of *Beng Lou*, the average number of *bao* administered were 11. The number of *bao* administered ranged between two and 36 per patient. 33 complete cures were obtained. In another 29 cases, clear improvement was apparent. In 11 others, some results were registered. And in 10 cases, no results were evident. These statistics yielded an 87.9% amelioration rate. TCM diagnoses for these 83 cases included Hot Blood, Stagnant Blood, Spleen Deficiency, Kidney Yang Deficiency, and Kidney Yin Deficiency. Since the clinical training available in Chinese medicine in the Unite States is generally not extensive, such figures are important to neophytes so that they in turn, can inform their patients of the probable parameters of their treatment in an honest and realistic way.

PREMENSTRUAL BREAST DISTENSION

A Precis and Commentary on
"Clinical Experience (in the treatment of) Premenstrual Breast Distention"
by Zhu Xiao-nan

Premenstrual breast distention, fibrocystic disease, and breast cancer are, from the point of view of Traditional Chinese Medicine, stages of a single continuum. At root, these problems are all due to Liver Qi Congestion. However, in individual patients, this may be complicated by any number of related disharmonies and, over time, this scenario may undergo transformation through certain progressions. The first two disorders named above respond very well to Traditional Chinese Medicine. Chinese-style treatment for them is typically successful in from three to four months. Even the third disorder, breast cancer, can often be treated successfully without recourse to surgery, radiation, or chemotherapy.

Shang Hai Lao Zhong Yi Jing Yan Xuan Bian (A Collection of Shanghai Old Masters' Clinical Experiences) is an anthology of monographs by contemporary Old Masters of Traditional Chinese Medicine in Shanghai.[1] In it, Zhu Xiao-nan gives a report on his experience with premenstrual breast distention. Zhu begins by stating that premenstrual breast distention is a commonly encountered complaint in clinical practice, yet there is scant mention of it in the medical classics. Zhu attributes this to two reasons. First, in the feudal society, doctors and patients did not discuss this problem out of modesty and fear. And secondly, when breast distention is associated with the period, it is a self-limiting symptoms and therefore its treatment is often overlooked. However, according to Zhu, it is a symptom to which attention should be paid. It is a hindrance to physical and mental well-being and it is associated with patterns of disharmony which can effect reproductive capacity and eventually systemic health. In Zhu Xiao-nan's experience, most Chinese women with premenstrual breast distention initiate TCM treatment for infertility. As we will discuss below, this is not the case with American patients.

Zhu Xiao-nan divides his essay, "Clinical Experience (in the treatment of) Premenstrual Breast Distention", into six sections plus a summary discussion. He begins in section one with an analysis of the symptoms of this disorder. According to him, in women who suffer from premenstrual breast distention, their breasts become swollen and tender three to ten days prior to the onset of the period. However, some women may experience discomfort at mid-cycle. I have even seen women who had breast distention three weeks out of every month. In most cases, the breast distention will disappear on its own on the first or second day of menstruation. Sometimes it will last through menstruation, but this is uncommon. The symptoms display a regular cyclic nature clearly associated with the menstrual cycle. The symptoms can be graded in four groups: simple breast distention, breast distention with pain in the nipple, distention with lumps, and lumps with inflammation.

In records of twenty Chinese women with breast distention, Zhu found that seventeen of them also experienced lower abdominal distention, low back pain, and dysmenorrhea. Ten of them also complained of poor appetite and/or indigestion.

168

Eight experienced chest oppression. Five had pain in their ovarian region. And four complained of lack of sexual desire. Eight of these patients had had Western gynecological exams. Three of the eight were diagnosed as having inflammation of the fallopian tubes. One had blocked tubes. Another had an underdeveloped uterus with inflammation of the tubes. A sixth had imperfect uterine development. The seventh had cervical inflammation. And the eighth had a loss of sensation in her genitalia. All twenty cases had a history of difficulty conceiving. Eleven out of twenty had not conceived in from two to five years. Six had not conceived in from six to ten years. And three had not conceived in from eleven to thirteen years.

Zhu's second section is a discussion of the five *Zheng* or patterns of disharmony in his experience responsible for the four, above-mentioned grades of breast disorder. They are Liver Qi Congestion with concomitant Spleen Deficiency, Liver Qi with Kidney Deficiency, Liver Qi with Blood Deficiency, Liver Qi with Deficiency Cold of the *Chong* and *Ren*, and Liver Qi with Fire Flaring. Zhu lists the signs and symptoms of each of these five *Zheng* as follows:

Liver Qi Congestion with Spleen Deficiency: premenstrual breast distention, chest oppression, decline in appetite, nausea, abdominal distention or a bearing down in the hypogastrium, and/or pain in the ovarian region. The pulse is typically wiry and fine. The tongue is pale and puffy with a thin white coat. To these symptoms I would add possible diarrhea, constipation, flatulence, belching, craving for sweets and carbohydrates, cold hands and feet, fatigue, and/or water retention. The exact constellation of symptoms will depend upon whether the Liver Qi or the Spleen Deficiency predominates. Furthermore, one must distinguish between Spleen Qi Deficiency and Spleen Yang Deficiency, although in American women Spleen Qi Deficiency, in my experience, is the more commonly

169

encountered. This scenario may also be frequently complicated in American women by Spleen Dampness.

Liver Qi with Kidney Deficiency: premenstrual breast distention, chest oppression, sore lower back, weak lower limbs, and a general lack of sexual desire. Typically the patient's menarche was late, i.e. between sixteen and twenty years of age. The tongue is pale with a scant coating and the pulse is most often deep and wiry. Zhu does not distinguish whether this is Kidney Qi, Kidney Yang, or Kidney *Jing* Deficiency. From the symptoms given it does not appear to be Kidney Yin Deficiency, and sexual desire is a function of Kidney Yang.

Liver Qi with Blood Deficiency: breast distention, dizziness, pale complexion, lengthened menstrual cycles, and scant menstrual discharge pale in color. The tongue is often purple with scant fur and the pulse is typically thready and wiry.

Liver Qi with Deficiency Cold of the *Chong* and *Ren*: breast distention, sore lower back, fatigue, a cold feeling in the lower abdomen. The tongue is pale with a thin white coat and the pulse is thready and slow.

Liver Qi with Fire Flaring: chest oppression, breast distention, dry mouth, Internal Heat, hypogastric pain or pain over the ovaries, and lower abdominal distention. Generally there is a turbid vaginal discharge. The tongue is pale red with a thin yellow coating. The pulse is wiry and a little fast. This could be either Excess Fire from transformed Stuck Qi or it could be Deficiency Fire due to Insufficient Yin. Herbal treatment would vary depending upon which of these two possibilities presented.

Zhu's third section is devoted to the herbal treatment of the above five *Zheng* and major accompanying symptoms. Zhu begins by giving a basic formula for activating the Qi, opening

170

Stagnation, strengthening the Spleen, and harmonizing the Stomach. Its ingredients are:

Rhizoma Cyperi	9 grams
Cortex Albizziae	9 "
Fructus Perillae	9 "
Fructus Liquidambaris	9 "
Tuber Curcumae	6 "
fried Rhizoma Atractylodis Macrocephalae	6 "
fried Radix Linderae	6 "
Pericarpium Citri Reticulatae	6 "
Fructus Citri Seu Ponciri Immaturi	6 "

This formula can then be modified in the following manner:

For breast distention, add Semen Citri Reticulatae and Folium Citri Reticulatae.

For breast distention with pain, add Fructus Meliae and Herba Cum Radice Taraxaci Mongolici.

For breast distention with lumps, add Semen Vaccariae and Squama Manitis.

For distention, lumps, and inflammation, add Herba Sargassi and Thallus Algae.

For Kidney Deficiency, add Cortex Eucommiae and Radix Dipsaci.

For Blood Deficiency, add Radix Angelicae Sinensis and Radix Rehmanniae Conquitae.

For Deficiency Cold of the *Chong* and *Ren*, add Colla Cornu Cervi and Cortex Cinnamomi.

For Flaring Fire, add Cortex Phellodendri and Herba Artemisiae Apiaciae.

For dragging pain over the ovaries, add Radix Pulsatillae and Caulis Sargentodoxae.

This is a very useful and effective formula. However, I would also like to add several other formulae to give the practitioner even more options. In the first three formulae, these additions will seem self-apparent, minor variation to those with a good working knowledge of Chinese medicinals. However, for beginners, it is useful to know that certain combinations have proven their effectiveness over time. The first formula is a variation of Chai Hu Shu Gan Tang (Bupleurum Liver Dredging Decoction). It is given by Xu Sheng-yang in *Qian Jia Miao Fang (A Thousand Practitioners' Wondrous Prescriptions)* [2] as an appropriate formula for a number of premenstrual disorders. Its ingredients are:

Radix Bupleuri	9 grams
Radix Angelicae Sinensis	12 "
Radix Paeoniae Albae	12 "
Tuber Curcumae	12 "
Fructus Citri Seu Ponciri Immaturi	9 "
Rhizoma Cyperi	9 "
Pericarpium Citri Reticulatae Viridis	9 "
Folium Citri Reticulatae	9 "
Fructus Liquidambaris	9 "

Xu Sheng-yang gives the following useful additions:

For irritability and Heat, add Cortex Radicis Moutan and Fructus Lycii.

For breast lumps, add Semen Vaccariae, Semen Citri

Reticulatae, and Melon Peduncle.

For headache, select from and add Fructus Viticis, Flos Chrysanthemi, Herba Menthae, Radix Angelicae, and/or Radix Puerariae.

For water retention, select from and add Rhizoma Atractylodis, Sclerotium Poriae Cocoris, and/or Semen Plantaginis.

For nipple or breast itchiness, select from and add Ramulus Uncariae Cum Uncis, Herba Seu Flos Schizonepetae, and/or Radix Ledebouriellae.

For vomiting, select from and add Caulis Bambusae In Taenium, Rhizoma Pinelliae, and/or Pericarpium Citri Seu Ponciri.

For Plum Seed Qi, add Cortex Magnoliae, Rhizoma Pinelliae, and Folium Perillae.

The second additional formula is for fibrocystic breast disease. It has been given by Cheung and Belluomini in "Traditional and New Interpretations of Prescriptions: The Harmonizing and Relieving Group".[3] Judging by its ingredients, it is for Stagnant Blood and Heat as well as Qi Congestion. It is a strong dispersing formula and it should only be given to patients robust enough and only for short periods of time. Its ingredients are:

Radix Bupleuri
Fructus Citri Seu Ponciri Immaturi
Pericarpium Citri Reticulatae Viridis
Rhizoma Acori Graminei
Rhizoma Cyperi
Tuber Curcumae

Radix Ligustici Wallichi
Radix Paeoniae Rubrae
Apex Radicis Angelicae Sinensis
Radix Rehmanniae
Semen Arecae
Gummi Olibanum
Concha Ostreae
Radix Glycyrrhizae
Herba Cum Radice Violae

One can also use the well-known Xiao Yao San (Free and Easy Powder) and modify it specifically to address breast distention. Its ingredients are:

Radix Bupleuri
Radix Angelicae Sinensis
Radix Paeoniae Albae
Rhizoma Atractylodis Macrocephalae
Scelrotium Poriae Cocoris
Radix Praeparatus Glycyrrhizae
Herba Menthae

To this basic formula, one may add for breast distention Semen Citri Reticulatae, Pericarpium Citri Reticulatae, and Pericarpium Viridis Citri Reticulatae. The basic formula is indicated for Liver Qi Congestion, Blood Deficiency, and Spleen Deficiency. It can be modified in many ways. A number of these modifications are given by Cheung and Belluomini.[4]

Since many American women suffer from Qi Congestion complicated by Yin Deficiency, care must be taken when using Qi-dispersing and Blood-dispersing herbs. In my experience, often Yin tonic herbs must be added to American women's prescriptions and the strength of the Qi-dispersing herbs modified. Or else, a course of Yin tonification after the period must counterbalance the Qi dispersion before the period.

And finally, a last formula which is useful in the treatment of mastoses is Shi Liu Wei Liu Chi Yin (Sixteen Flavored Flowing Qi Drink). Hsu Hong-yen lists among its indications fibrocystic disease, breast cancer, and intraductal papillomas. This formula was originally included in the carbuncle section of the Ming dynasty *Wan Ping Hui Chun*. Hsu and Hsu state it "is used for treating a severe abscess of unknown etiology, carbuncles, and breast cancer...(it) is suitable for disintegrating unknown toxic tumors."[5] Although this formula contains a number of Qi-regulating and dispersing ingredients, it also tonifies the Qi and Blood and therefore it can be used over a longer period of time or in rotation with more dispersing formulae. I have used this formula successfully in the case of severe fibrocystic disease. Its ingredients are:

> Radix Angelicae Sinensis
> Cortex Cinnamomi
> Radix Platycodi
> Radix Linderae
> Semen Arecae
> Radix Ligustici Wallichi
> Radix Codonopsis Pilosulae
> Radix Astragali Seu Hedysari
> Cortex Magnoliae
> Fructus Perillae
> Radix Paeoniae Albae
> Radix Angelicae
> Radix Saussureae Seu Vladimiriae
> Fructus Citri Seu Ponciri Immaturi
> Radix Ledebouriellae
> Radix Glycyrrhizae

Zhu Xiao-nan does not mention acupuncture in his article.

However, acupuncture protocols can be easily created for each of the five *Zheng* discussed above and the major presenting symptoms. In my experience, acupuncture is a useful adjunctive therapy in the treatment of premenstrual breast distention and other mastoses. It is not unusual for the patient to notice significant decrease in distention and tenderness immediately after an acupuncture treatment. Yuan Shou, Zhang Yu-hua, and Kang Xiu-sheng suggest a basic protocol consisting of the local points *Ru Gen* (St 18), *Yin Chuang* (St 16), *Shang Zhong* (CV 17), and *Qi Men* (Liv 14) for mastoses in general.[6] To such local points may be added the following distal points which, in my opinion, will make the treatment even more effective:

For breast distention, add *Liang Qiu* (St. 34), the *Xi* Cleft point of the Foot *Yang Ming*.

For nipple pain, add *Xing Jian* (Liv 2), the Sedation point of the Foot *Jue Yin*.

For Liver Qi, add *Nei Guan* (Per 6), *Tai Chong* (Liv 3), and/or *San Yin Jiao* (Sp 6).

For Liver Fire, needle *Xing Jian* instead of *Tai Chong*.

For Kidney Deficiency, add *Tai Xi* (Ki 3) and *Shen Shu* (Bl 23).

For Deficiency Cold of the *Chong* and *Ren*, moxa *Guan Yuan* (CV 4).

For Flaring Fire, add *Lao Gong* (Per 8), *Xin Shu* (Bl 15), and *Tai Xi*.

For Stagnant Blood in the breast with pricking pain through to the back, add *Ge Shu* (Bl 17), *Jue Yin Shu* (Bl 14), and *Xin*

Shu.

For Phlegm obstructing the *Jing Luo*, add *Zu San Li* (St 36) and *Feng Long* (St 40).

Indirect moxa on ginger directly over any lumps and/or ginger compresses are also useful adjunctive therapies. Compresses can be done by the patient at home. They help to involve the patient in her treatment and return some of the responsibility for her health back to her.

Likewise, Zhu Xiao-nan also does not discuss diet or lifestyle modifications. Both of these are, in my experience, vitally important in achieving a lasting treatment for this and related disorders. I have discussed these issues vis a vis Liver Congestion at length elsewhere.[7] However, briefly, the patient should be encouraged to avoid coffee *completely*, both caffeinated and decaff. She should also cut down on spicy, greasy, oily, and sour foods and alcohol. Most importantly, she should be carefully advised about proper exercise and stress reduction.

Zhu's fourth section is comprised of further instructions in his treatment plan. Basically, he suggests beginning treatment when the breast distention presents each month. Treatment should continue until the symptoms abate. This constitutes one course of treatment and typically there should be clear and distinct results in three to four courses, i.e. three to four menstrual cycles. This, likewise, is my experience. However, I would also suggest continuing treatment in a modified form between periods. This can be done with Xiao Yao Wan, Ba Zhen Wan, Shu Gan Wan, or other appropriate patent pills. More than one prescription can be combined to fit the patient's Root disharmony. Our stress, unlike Chinese, is continuous, unrelenting, and unrelieved. American women, in my experience, need more external support and treatment than their Chinese counterparts. Criteria for deciding on such background treatment should be based on traditional Chinese pathophysiology and the patient's immediate diagnosis during the various phases of her cycle.

In section five, Zhu gives the results of treating the above-mentioned twenty women. Of the twenty, the smallest number of packets or *bao* was three. The largest was forty-one. The average was ten. After successful treatment, i.e. relief of the breast distention and accompanying symptoms, thirteen women conceived. Six women experienced subjective improvement but did not conceive. Only one patient reported no results or improvements. Of the fourteen women suffering from Liver Qi and Spleen Deficiency, there were eleven cures and ten pregnancies. Three other cases improved. Of the three cases of Liver Qi and Kidney Deficiency, two improved and one showed no result. There was one example each of the other three *Zheng* and of these, all were cured and all became pregnant.

In section six, Zhu Xiao-nan gives three case histories. However, instead of reporting on these I would like to give one of my own, since, for American practitioners, American case histories are more germane. The patient was thirty-two year old. She was a single mother of a four year old son. In addition, she was going to school to learn a new profession. Her major complaint was PMS. She complained of being angry of late. Two weeks before, she had been depressed over the Christmas holidays. She experienced some pain under her ribs on the right side after drinking coffee. Recently she had been experiencing premenstrual breast distention and soreness. She also had Plum Seed Qi which an MD had diagnosed as a benign growth inside of her throat. Her cycle was regular at twenty-eight days but scant. Her sleep was good. She reported that her bowel movements were normal, although she mentioned she had a movement after every meal. However, when asked if her stools tended to be loose, she said that they were well formed. The patient had had three abortions eight to twelve years previously. She had herpes genitalia but her outbreaks were infrequent. She also had recurrent yeast infections which caused vaginal pruritus accompanied by a pale yellow, creamy discharge. Her tongue was normal except for a red tip. The coating was clear white. Her pulse was somewhat slippery on the right. The patient said that she had had a cup of coffee just before the appointment. On the left, her pulse was wiry in the *Chi* position. My diagnosis was Liver Qi Congestion with possible Spleen Deficiency. My assumption was that, during times of additional stress, the congestion transformed into Fire. I prescribed a modified Chai Hu Shu Gan Tang:

Radix Bupleuri	9 grams
Radix Paeoniae Albae	12 "
Radix Angelicae Sinensis	12 "
Fructus Citri Seu Ponciri Immaturi	9 "
Radix Achyranthis	9 "
Rhizoma Cyperi	9 "
Tuber Curcumae	12 "
Pericarpium Viridis Citri Reticulatae	9 "
Folium Perillae	9 "

The patient took four *bao* of this formula the first month preceding her period. She reported complete relief of her breast distention and soreness within two days. She also experienced more emotional stability and less irritability. The next cycle, she took the same formula with similar good results. The third cycle the patient reported that her stools had become long and skinny and not as complete feeling. Therefore, I added 9 grams each of Sclerotium Poriae Cocoris and Rhizoma Atractylodis Macrocephalae, which remedied the situation. After three cycles the patient felt she did not need

179

any further herbal treatment. However, she did continue with the dietary modifications, including complete abstinence from coffee, a twenty minute per day deep relaxation practice, and regular exercise. I do not know if the Plum Seed Qi changed or improved. My guess is that a different formula more specific for that condition would be needed to address that problem. Since an MD had diagnosed a growth, it is very likely that the patient felt it was not a condition amenable to traditional Chinese therapy.

Following these six sections, Zhu Xiao-nan ends with a general discussion of the relevant traditional theories which account for premenstrual breast distention. Zhu says that the primary factor in this condition is Liver Qi Congestion. Due to emotional excess, anger, frustration, and stress, the Liver Qi loses its free flowing patency. This results in Excess Qi in the Liver which vents on or invades the Stomach through the *Ke* cycle of Five Phase theory. Therefore, there is simultaneous disturbance, i.e. Congestion, in both the Foot *Jue Yin* and the Foot *Yang Ming* meridians. The nipple is under the control of the Liver, while the breast is under the Stomach. Nipple pain and breast distention are examples of this mutual involvement between these two organs. Zhu emphasizes this close connection between stuck and knotted Liver Qi and breast distention. He recounts a story of a woman who had premenstrual breast distention. Once, during mid-cycle when her breasts were otherwise not sore or distended, she became very angry and upset. Immediately her breasts swelled up and became sore just as if she were premenstrual. This is Zhu's way of stressing the importance of psychoemotional factors in this disorder.

The Liver meridian traverses the reproductive organs. Problems in the reproductive organs are often related to or caused by Liver disharmony. The *Ren Mai* circulates inside the abdomen. It rules conception. The *Ren Mai* and the Liver meridian have a very close relationship. Their Channels run along the same path in the hypogastrium and they have common meeting points at *Qu Gu* (CV 2), *Zhong Ji* (CV 3), and *Guan Yuan*. When the menses is just about due, the Sea of Blood is full and there may be tenderness in the hypogastrium. Therefore, if there is Liver Qi Congestion, it will be aggravated and consequently will display clear symptoms at this time. Above there will be chest oppression and breast distention and below there will be hypogastric pain and distention.

After the menstrual flow begins, the Sea of Blood gradually empties. Therefore, the tender feeling diminishes. The Liver Stagnation softens and harmonizes and the breast and abdominal distention are levelled. This cycle repeats itself over and over again. After some time, this may lead to an inability to conceive.

While treating this problem, Zhu says to begin when the distention begins and to suspend treatment when it dissipates. Continue this way for three to four months and you will get very clear results. Often patients will not experience pain or distention every month. In my opinion, this is most often due to the alternating activity of the ovaries. Stagnation of the Liver meridian may be primarily located on one side of the hypogastrium. Another cause for this break in cyclicity might also be fluctuations in stress, exercise, and diet. If such women consider themselves cured and therefore do not take any further herbal medicine, the next month their symptoms will return and unfortunately will have to begin treatment over again.

Zhu wrote his essay for other Chinese clinicians. American practitioners of Traditional Chinese Medicine generally are not as extensively schooled and thoroughly trained as their Chinese counterparts. Therefore, I believe some further clarification

181

of Chinese medical theory vis a vis the menstruation is appropriate. According to Chinese theory, the mechanism of menstruation is regulated by the proper functioning of the *Chong* and *Ren*. The *Chong* is the Sea of Blood and Blood is the material basis of the menstruation. The *Ren* governs the patency of Qi and therefore regulates the flow of the menstruation. Qi and Blood relate to Yang and Yin respectively. At the onset of the period, the *Chong* and *Ren* are both replete and functioning at maximum activity. During the period there is a loss or discharge of Blood. At the end of this period, the *Chong* is relatively Blood Deficient. Since the Blood is a species of Yin, if there is systemic Yin Deficiency, there will be some difficulty replenishing the Blood and *Chong*. This may cause or aggravate Yin Deficiency symptoms at this time. During the week following the cessation of menstruation, the Kidneys, which store the *Jing*, and the Liver, which stores the Blood, are called upon to replenish this Deficiency. During the next week, corresponding to mid-cycle, the *Chong* and *Ren* are again at peak activity, which is why some women experience mid-cycle abdominal cramping. Whereas during the first week after menstruation the Yin and Blood were growing, now the Yang and Qi grow for the next week.

At this point, i.e. one week before the onset of the period, this Yang Qi must flow down below the *Dai Mai* in order to activate the Blood accumulating in the pelvis and discharge it. However, since Yang Qi tends to float upwards, if the Liver's dredging function is impaired, this Qi may not flow down into the pelvis. If instead this Qi inappropriately accumulates in the upper half of the body, there may be chest oppression, breast distention, headaches, including migraines, and emotional lability. If the passages which direct the flow of Yang Qi downwards, primarily the Eight Extraordinary meridians, are unblocked and functioning correctly, these symptoms will not appear and the menstruation will proceed normally. That is

182

why, in several of the formulae given for premenstrual breast distention, there are ingredients specifically to lead this Qi downward, such as Radix Achyranthes and Fructus Perillae. Informed treatment for menstrual disorders, whether with herbs or acupuncture, should take these four seven day phases of the menstrual cycle into account for maximum efficiency.

Although I think Zhu Xiao-nan's entire article and his summary discussion of premenstrual breast distention are quite good, I believe there are a few additional points that are necessary to mention in terms of American patients. First, unlike Chinese women who want to conceive, I believe many American women in their thirties develop this problem because they have consciously avoided conception or limited it to only one child relatively early in their child-bearing years. Child-bearing is a larger version of the monthly menstrual discharge which can have profound harmonizing effects on the *Jue Yin*, Sea of Blood, *Ren Mai* and *Chong Mai*. Likewise, suckling is what the breasts have been created for, and suckling is good for the breast tissue. Abortions, pelvic infections due to IUDs, and tubal ligations tend to cause or aggravate Stagnation in the pelvis and therefore in the *Jue Yin* whose duty it is to maintain the patency of Qi. These factors are further complicated by the incompletely and erroneously treated sequelae of vaginal and urinary infections and venereal disease.

Furthermore, American women today are under historically unique and unrelieved stresses. Added to the generally frenetic and stressful pace of modern life in the West, women are also subjected to the burdens of single parenthood, multiple and poorly defined roles, the pressures of dating and the continual sexual decisions and anxieties which attend to that, economic discrimination, and lack of extended family and communal support. Liver Qi Congestion is primarily due to emotional frustration, and contemporary American women find themselves in a myriad of situation where they are damned if

183

they do and damned if they don't.

It is my belief that the practitioner should try to help his or her patients understand the social and emotional factors which have led to an epidemic incidence of Liver Qi Congestion in American women. Although each of us bears responsibility for our own lives, taking responsibility begins with recognition of the forces and factors to which we are subject. By helping patients to more clearly see the factors responsible for their frustration, they will, in most cases, feel less frustrated rather than more. Although our world and society are not going to change overnight, skillfully managing one's lifestyle, stress, exercise, and diet can go a long way in mitigating the ill-effects of our modern environment. Since subjective and objective realities are coterminous, inseparable, and relatively interdependent, each time we alter our perception of our situation, i.e. our own mind, we alter the world in which we find ourselves.

ENDNOTES

1   *Shang Hai Lao Zhong Yi Jing Yan Xuan Bian*, ed.
     Shanghai Municipal Health Office, (Shanghai Science
     and Technology Press), Shanghai, PRC, 1984

2   *Qian Jia Miao Fang*, ed. Li Wen-liang, Qi Qiang, et.al.,
     (Liberation Army Publishing), Beijing, 1985, p. 13-15

3   Cheung, C.S. & Belluomini, Jenny, "Traditional and
     New Interpretations of Prescriptions: The Harmonizing
     and Relieving Group", *Journal of Amer. Coll. of TCM*,
     San Francisco, #1, 1984, p. 10 & 11

4   Ibid., p. 8 - 11

5   Hsu Hong-yen & Hsu Chau-shin, *Commonly Used
     Chinese Herb Formulas with Illustrations*, (OHAI), LA,
     1980, p. 403

6   Yuan Shou, Zhang Yu-hua, & Kang Xin-sheng, "110
     Cases of Mastosis Treated by Acupuncture", *Journal of
     Chinese Medicine*, UK, #19, Sept. 1985, p. 26 & 27

7   Flaws, Bob, "Premenstrual Syndrome (PMS): Its
     Differential Diagnosis and Treatment", *American
     Journal of Acupuncture*, Felton, CA, Vol. 13, #3, Sept.
     1985, p. 205-222

8   Ross, Jeremy, "Traditional Chinese Medicine and
     Gynaecology, Part One", *Journal of Chinese Medicine*,
     UK, #11, Jan. 1983, p. 18 & 19

OTHER BOOKS ON CHINESE MEDICINE
AVAILABLE FROM
BLUE POPPY PRESS

MIGRAINES & TRADITIONAL CHINESE MEDICINE: A Layperson's Guide by Bob Flaws ISBN 0-936185-15-5 $11.95

ENDOMETRIOSIS & INFERTILITY AND TRADITIONAL CHINESE MEDICINE: A Laywoman's Guide by Bob Flaws ISBN 0-936185-14-7 $9.95

CLASSICAL MOXIBUSTION SKILLS IN CONTEMPORARY CLINICAL PRACTICE by Sung Baek ISBN 0-936185-16-3 $10.95

THE BREAST CONNECTION: A Laywoman's Guide to the Treatment of Breast Disease by Chinese Medicine
by Honora Lee Wolfe ISBN 0-936185-13-9 $8.95

NINE OUNCES: A Nine Part Program For The Prevention of AIDS in HIV Positive Persons by Bob Flaws ISBN 0-936185-12-0 $8.95

THE TREATMENT OF CANCER BY INTEGRATED CHINESE-WESTERN MEDICINE by Zhang Dai-zhao, trans. by Zhang Ting-liang & Bob Flaws, ISBN 0-936185-11-2 $16.95

BLUE POPPY ESSAYS: 1988 Translations and Ruminations on Chinese Medicine by Bob Flaws, et al, ISBN 0-936185-10-4 $18.95

A HANDBOOK OF TRADITIONAL CHINESE DERMATOLOGY by Liang Jian-hui, trans. by Zhang Ting-liang & Bob Flaws, ISBN 0-936185-07-4 $14.95

SECRET SHAOLIN FORMULAE FOR THE TREATMENT OF EXTERNAL INJURY by Patriarch De Chan, trans. by Zhang Ting-liang & Bob Flaws, ISBN 0-936185-08-2 $12.95

A HANDBOOK OF TRADITIONAL CHINESE GYNECOLOGY by Zhejiang College of TCM, trans. by Zhang Ting-liang, ISBN 0-936185-06-6 $17.95

FREE & EASY: Traditional Chinese Gynecology for American Women by Bob Flaws, ISBN 0-936185-05-8 $15.95

PRINCE WEN HUI'S COOK: Chinese Dietary Therapy by Bob Flaws & Honora Lee Wolfe, ISBN 0-912111-05-4, $12.95 (Published by Paradigm Press, Brookline, MA)

TURTLE TAIL & OTHER TENDER MERCIES: Traditional Chinese Pediatrics by Bob Flaws ISBN 0-936185-00-7 $14.95